LIFE IN 20 LESSONS

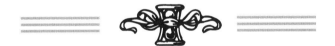

What a Funeral Guy Discovered about Life, from Death

CHRIS MEYER

Life in 20 Lessons
© 2020 Chris Meyer

ISBN (print, soft cover): 978-1-7333443-0-2
ISBN (print, hard cover): 978-1-7333443-1-9
ISBN (ebook): 978-1-7333443-2-6
ISBN (audiobook): 978-1-7333443-3-3

Book design and production: www.DominiDragoone.com
Editorial: Sandra Wendel, Write On, Inc.
Audio Book: edited and mixed by David Whitaker at Post Audio Eureka, CA
Author photo © Kendra Malek

Published by
Meaning of Life Publishing
ChrisMeyerAuthor.com

Contents

DEDICATION

To my parents…The greatest parents a child could ever ask for. Period. End of story. You have given me everything, and so much more. I will pay it forward.

And to my wife…What do I say? Simply, my everything.

To my brothers who left this earth too soon: Tony, Ned, and TJ. I have the memories.

Author Disclaimer

I speak of God in this book.

I grew up going to an evangelical Lutheran church (the less strict kind) most every Sunday of my childhood. After graduating from high school, I never went to church regularly again. While I am not what a layman would describe as religious, I do believe in a Higher Power—and an afterlife.

Seeing what I have seen after a career in the funeral industry might make you a believer too.

When I speak of my Higher Power in the few instances in this book, please simply insert whomever, or whatever, you believe in, if anything. In my world, one is not better than the other; it is simply in what/whom you choose to believe. I believe all of our Higher Powers would respect each other's right to choose. At least that's how I want to go through life. Whomever bless you.

Introduction

As a man over fifty years of age, statistically, I have lived more than half of my life.

For the last fourteen years of that life, I have owned a funeral home. It has taught me the most about the human condition and myself. I have seen horrific, absolutely horrific, things, smelled smells that are unimaginable, cried with friends and strangers, and witnessed unspeakable tragedy, heartache, and death all too often for one human being.

But the funeral home has also given me my greatest gift—perspective. If you think your day is going badly, someone always has it worse, way worse, guaranteed.

You've heard it all before: Each day above ground is a blessing, live each day as if it were your last, or any one of the manifold great quotes about being alive.

They are all true.

And now, in some way, I can see there may have been a purpose to all this. Like maybe I was meant to be a conduit, of sorts, between the surviving and the dead.

I have sat with the survivors. I have listened to their stories, their cries, their confessions, their regrets, their wishes, their "would'ves," "should'ves," and "could'ves." I have just closed my mouth and listened.

In listening to the survivors, I have heard the dead. Not in any creepy M. Night Shyamalan "I see dead people" type of way, but in being around so much death, listening to families and loved ones' stories, eulogies, services, pastors, preachers, passages, and musical selections, I have gained some insights over the years, some expertise.

And, for me, the bonus was that I raised a family just as I started in the funeral industry. Our lives together became the test case for the lessons I was learning about life, from death. After seeing the impact on my own family, I knew I could help a lot of people with this information.

So I sat down and memorialized the lessons I learned to make certain you don't search your whole life only to realize the true meaning of life on your deathbed.

But make no mistake, this is not a funeral book. This is a story of living—with "insider's knowledge." Sure, I will tell you funeral stories from where I drew inspiration. That is my platform, the reason you should listen to me, why I am an "expert in the field"—at least that is what the publishers and editors have told me.

Fair enough.

But, honestly, there is as much inspiration from my current and past lives herein. Because I am not only a funeral guy, but also a father, a husband, a son, a grandson, a brother, a coach, and a friend.

In the end, this is not a funeral story. This is story about how one man discovered life in the funeral business…by living death.

1 Be Thankful

PATTY

The front door opened at the funeral home, like it had a thousand times before, and in walked a husband and wife. They were clearly looking around, as people often do, judging the cleanliness, the creepiness, the overall complexion of this, admittedly, scary place to enter.

By this time in my career, I was used to their wariness and tried to let my patrons do their thing until I could tell they wanted my help. I had owned the funeral home in Northern California for more than five years at that point. I was slowly getting more comfortable in my role.

As they walked closer, the woman's face came into focus. The side of her face was slumped as if she had had a stroke and one eye was half open.

"May I help you?" I asked with a smile.

"Yes. We would like to discuss funeral arrangements."

"For Mom, Dad, a grandparent?"

"For me," she said.

I stared into her eyes. This had never happened to me before—a person with a few months to live, planning their own funeral.

And so began a funeral arrangement that would change my world forever.

Her name was Patty. She was not quite fifty, a small, cherubic-looking woman with large glasses. I found out she was told she had a few months to live. She had two children, whom she loved very much, and a husband, Bruce (with her), whom she said "could not handle these types of ordeals." She meant no disrespect in her comment, and her husband clearly took no offense. She knew she had to handle this for him, so he would be okay. A selfless act of love.

And she was right. Bruce just looked right through me with a blank, glossed-over death stare, as if to say "my wife is going to die soon."

Patty asked me a litany of questions (Who will come and get me? Where will I go? How soon after I die will the cremation take place? When can my family pick up my remains and take me home?), all of which I had been asked a hundred times before. I always try to tailor my message to each family, but in this case to Patty herself. I could see the deliberate nods of her head as I answered each question, all the while never taking her eyes off mine, staying with me, looking more deeply, almost through me.

Her husband, meanwhile, stared straight at the floor, clearly in shock at the enormity of what lay ahead for him and his children— as many of us men would do, thinking of parenting the rest of our lives without our clearly better halves.

After I had gone through the process, she continued to look at me and I at her. She stared into my eyes for what seemed like an eternity. I never left her stare. I could see her mind processing. I could see her evaluating me: Is this guy for real? Is he sincere? Does he really mean what he is saying or is this just another arrangement?

I see it. I see each question unfolding in her eyes. Then, she said, "I've been to a lot of places."

I nod my understanding.

"I want you to take care of me."

"I would be honored," I replied.

And with that, Patty, her husband, and I planned her funeral.

She told me about her children, what she wanted for each of them and for their lives, what she wanted for her husband in her passing, what she wanted for the family when she was gone. There was so much grace in her words. So much dignity. So much strength. My God, the strength of this woman. It exuded from her every pore.

As I looked at Patty, all I could think of was my two boys and my third on the way. What if this was my wife, or me, with a life ahead to live with our children without the other one of us?

Patty just kept staring at me, her face slumped on one side from that insidious tumor in her head, but her chin raised, dignified, powerful, strong in her weakness.

Months went by until I got the call.

"Chris, they requested you."

This happens sometimes with friends' families. But I didn't recognize the name, at first. It wasn't until I saw her husband at the front door of their home that I knew. We embraced.

When I stepped inside, I immediately saw her. There was Patty, in a hospital bed, in the middle of the living room. Patty was half the woman she was when she had walked into my funeral home just a few short months earlier. The brain cancer had changed her face. Her complexion was now the jaundiced yellow of organs shutting down, and her body was thin and frail, the result of her protracted illness.

What was undeniably apparent in this living room was the love this woman had been surrounded by, inundated with, in these last few months of her life: photos of her children as babies, growing up, as teenagers, some with Mom and Dad, some without. Handwritten cards, the ones that really matter in which people truly share their innermost feelings. A few scattered vases with flowers, a selection of stuffed animals: a bear, a dog, and a hippo. It was comfort, it was tranquility, it was love.

You see, Patty knew she was going to die. She knew it wouldn't be long. But if she was going to die, she wanted it to be the way *she* wanted it to be, in her home, surrounded by her children, her husband, her family, comfort, and love—a ton of love.

I bit the inside of my mouth to hold back tears as her children watched me kneel down to take their mother; they didn't know of our connection from the months prior and tears wouldn't be professional. Maneuvering around the medicine bottles, boxes of Kleenex, Gatorade, and unfinished plates of food, I lifted the hand-crocheted afghan off her and gently moved her to our collapsible cot.

I did what I had to do and took her back to the funeral home. I said a prayer with her, for her, and prayed for her husband and their family too.

I was thankful I met Patty. It was horrible that it was under those circumstances, but that was my vocation. Patty showed me how to live by letting me arrange her funeral that day. And while she never came out and said it, the way Patty looked at me told me everything I needed to know.

Never forsake even one day with your loved ones, for you know not what tomorrow will bring.

And she showed me how to spend our last days, surrounded by love. I know she would've wanted me to share that with you. On that day, Patty reconfirmed that love and family are the only answer. What else is there?

I am thankful Patty chose me, in life, to take care of her, in death.

MR. DOVI

Mr. Dovi was a father in our town when I was growing up. His son was a year younger than I, and Mr. Dovi would coach us in a variety of sports in third through eighth grade. He took time away from his job so he could coach. He was an inspiring coach, always stressing fundamentals, and he would get out there and participate too. You could tell he was having fun, and all of us kids loved it.

If you had Mr. Dovi as a coach, you were gonna have a good season.

I was a pretty good athlete for my age, and I genuinely loved playing sports. My parents never had to do anything to get me ready. I can distinctly remember getting up at the crack of dawn every Saturday because of my excitement for a baseball game, getting myself breakfast, and paying a religious-like attention to putting on my uniform a certain way, pulling the stirrups up high (ya know, style points).

I would walk to the field because my parents and brothers were usually still asleep. And I was always the first one there. I would sit in the vacant stands, listen to the birds chirping, smell the freshly cut grass, and enjoy the serenity of the vacant field. I look back on those days with fondness and clearly remember my love of the game (whatever the season).

And I was the kind of kid any coach would love. I never missed a practice and went hard whether it was a game or practice. I truly loved playing sports, which was ironic because my father was not particularly athletic, never once encouraged me to play anything, and was usually working long and hard to provide for our family.

Mr. Dovi coached me on and off from third through eighth grade, those magical years. And he liked me. His son Joey and I had a nice friendship besides being in different grades. I can distinctly remember Mr. Dovi pulling me aside after our last football game in sixth grade, placing his arm on my shoulder, looking deep into my eyes, and telling me, "I hope my boy grows up to be like you one day." (I was not even a year older than his son at the time.)

Pretty heady stuff for a sixth-grader to hear. He meant it too.

I had always liked Mr. Dovi, but hearing those compliments from him made him even more special in my eyes. I respected him for what he did for the boys of our community; he gave a part of himself, his time, for all of us. And he never got paid, in cash, for that time.

I know now, clearer than ever, that memories were his currency of choice.

After college I tracked him down at his house and sat with him for an hour. I wanted to tell him how much it meant to me to hear those words that day in sixth grade but, even more so, I wanted to thank him for coaching all of us boys, all those years.

He was humble and not really sure how to react. To him, I think, coaching was simply what he loved to do, and to be with his son and his son's friends. To me, it was the impact he made not only on me, but on our entire community. He took the time out of his day to provide us with instruction, mentoring, and guidance in our formative years. Sure, he liked to win, we all did, but deep down he just wanted us to improve and have fun.

When I moved to California, he got sick and, after a long illness, passed away. I wrote a note to his wife telling her of my love and appreciation for her husband.

I often thought, where was Mr. Dovi's participation trophy for all that he did? Where was his "extra few years card" from Our Maker for impacting the lives of countless young boys in our community?

Did he know how much we appreciated him? Did he well up with pride from all that coaching? I suspect he had the memories in his heart and mind. And, hopefully, there were reminders from guys like his son and me telling him how thankful we were.

I was lucky. I was really lucky to have a man like Tony Dovi to coach and love our community like I know he did. He inspired me to be present and coach everything I could possibly coach for each of my sons and their friends.

They are only young once.

COACHING AS AN EXCUSE

I have carried Mr. Dovi's inspiration into my own life with my sons. I have coached them all in a variety of sports: soccer, basketball, flag football—whatever they play. I love it, not because I love coaching, but because I too enjoy being with my sons and their friends. You get to learn so much about them. The fun we share, the laughs, the talks about teams and competitors, it is like no other for me. I get so much more than I give.

I would say I am not a particularly great strategist, but I am a solid teacher of fundamentals, a sound motivator, and good at defining roles each child can play to make our team better. I always stress the love of defense and not caring who scores, which is a difficult lesson when everyone just wants to score. I never talk about statistics at the end of the game, but rather how we did defensively. If we prevent baskets, we do not need to score as much.

For me, it has been an enlightening study in human behavior to see where a child is in the birth order of his family, if he has brothers or sisters, if his parents are married or divorced—all these aspects play a part in the psychology of coaching. Sure, we want to have fun and win, but you must tailor your coaching to each child's needs. At least that's how Mr. Dovi taught me.

There are kids who cry all the time, kids who fear nothing, kids who can't handle pressure, kids who love the game, and kids who are there because their moms just want them to be part of something in hopes of igniting the currently fluttering spark of enthusiasm for anything that is not a video game.

To me, it doesn't matter.

I am particularly lucky to be able to coach at my sons' school. They need coaches, and various moms and dads perform this function with joy. In my case, I have been coaching my sons' friends since they were in kindergarten. After all these years, you grow up with them and they become so much more than your sons' friends.

My middle son's friends are a particularly competitive group of boys who have had a lot of success. One year, when they were in fifth grade playing against sixth graders, they had a particularly good run. Even though they were the younger kids, they were beating most of the sixth-grade teams. In fact, we beat one team three separate times and then had a scheduled date to meet them in the semifinals of our league basketball championship.

We practiced the same, added a few nuances, and were totally ready for the game. And we lost.

The boys were shattered. Most of them were crying, totally inconsolable. I gave what I considered a legendary Wooden-esque speech of going down fighting and laying it all on the floor, before I told them how proud I was of the way they played, not only in that game, but the entire season. I was sweating and on the verge of tears myself.

It didn't help. There were tears everywhere, except for this one kid in the corner. He just kept looking up at me with a straight face.

I gave everyone a hug or a pat on the back as we left the hallway of the gym when I noticed this kid smiling as he was coming toward me. I looked at him and asked, "You okay?" expecting to hear his extreme sadness of the dream season vanquished before his eyes.

Without missing a beat, he snickered at me and said, "It's fifth-grade basketball, Coach."

From the mouths of babes.

I have received way more than I have ever given by coaching children. And, for me, it is really just an excuse to be with my sons and their friends in a setting other than playing at home.

I now clearly see what Mr. Dovi obviously knew in his heart all those years ago. I am thankful I have had the opportunity to play a small part in some children's lives. As I am writing this book, I have been blessed to have multiple players do presentations about me for their chapel public speaking exercises. I am humbled, honored, thankful. Coaching is among my most cherished days.

IN SUM

When you spend time in the funeral industry, you could go one of two ways: start drinking at 10:34 a.m. each day to dampen the demons of dealing with death or become thankful for even the smallest things in life. I chose the latter. Meeting with people in their time of need changed my world forever. It forced me to reflect on life, and on the people in it, and reminded me of what is truly important. The gift of working in the funeral industry can never be repaid.

Think of the people who impact your life today and thank them.

You will see that it makes you both feel good. Don't hold back because you think it might be awkward. Take the chance while they are alive to tell them what they have meant to you. I am telling you firsthand. I have seen too many people at graveside services or in eulogies say, "I wish I would have told them when they were alive. If only I had one more chance. Just one more chance."

This is it. Right here, right now. Tell them how they have touched your life. You will remember that moment forever and feel thankful that you took the time after they are gone.

Nothing bad comes from saying thank you.

THE REMINDERS

Be thankful for all that today brings.

———————————

Death is the greatest reminder of how to live or start living your own life.

———————————

Giving your time to your children and their friends will change lives.

———————————

2 Make a Difference

She was outside the house as I pulled up. I stepped out of the Honda Odyssey in which the rear seats had been replaced by a tray on which a collapsible cot sits—our funeral home's removal vehicle. As I walked toward the home, Cindy greeted me.

"We've got a false positive," she said.

"A false positive?"

"Not dead yet. They jumped the gun."

I am from the funeral home. Cindy is the hospice worker. I was called before she was. The person was not actually dead. The family thought their loved one had passed and jumped the gun because they did not know the protocol of calling the hospice worker first (once hospice pronounces the person's death, they instruct the family to call a funeral home). Now, I had to go home.

Cindy apologized profusely.

I smiled. She knew. This is one you don't get paid for. This trip was gratis. You can't bill the family for a false positive.

Hospice workers like Cindy are amazing people. They come in all shapes and sizes but are traditionally women with a calling.

They come into our lives when people wish to die at home and be kept comfortable. They are called in when there is simply precious little time left, generally under six months to live.

They administer drugs to keep a patient comfortable as they near death, so they don't suffer. I have been to many homes when a family member can't leave and yet they want to take care of a loved one's funeral. Invariably I am there with hospice, and we coordinate our services accordingly.

To me, hospice workers are some of the true angels of this earth. They are the most compassionate, knowledgeable, most caring people for the end-of-life journey. It is as if they have a sixth sense. And most people are unaware of the resource they provide at or near the end of life. Hospice workers make a huge difference in this world.

I had met Cindy before. In this moment of levity, I asked her why she does what she does. It's obviously not for the pay. It's obviously not for the light, cheery nature of the clientele or their situation. It's a calling.

In my limited experience with hospice, I think they were inspired by someone who treated them with dignity and respect during an end-of-life situation in their life or because they genuinely feel they can help other people at the worst time of their lives.

Believe it or not there are people who gravitate to these situations.

In Cindy's case it was the way her own mother was treated by hospice as she was dying. Cindy explained that she watched these people come in and out of her house at various times of the day and night, and yet treat her mother as if she were the only one who mattered and not like they had four other cases prior and two more homes to visit. And in many of these situations, they were volunteers; they were not even paid.

Think of the type of person who is drawn to that calling. Cindy was such a person. She was goodness personified. And she is one of many. Hospice workers make a difference.

THE EXPONENTIAL IMPACT OF COLLECTIVE GOODNESS

The world is a vast place. Your impact does not have to be world wide or epic. If we all start small, locally, and make a difference in our own community, it will compound exponentially and sprout the world-changing leaders of tomorrow: the Gandhis, the Mother Teresas, the Gateses, and so on.

But larger-than-life, world-changing leaders aside, altruism is happening daily, on a micro level, right here in our own communities. I am talking about the vast numbers of people doing simple good deeds and acts of kindness, the bulk of which we never hear about in the news: soup kitchens, food pantries, church groups, Kiwanis, Elks Clubs, volunteers, parents at schools, social workers, teachers, and the like. The examples are endless.

I see such volunteerism in my community, and there are thousands, millions of others making a difference and receiving no recognition for it around the globe. When you see these acts of kindness and compassion, stop them and simply say thank you. You will not believe how this will make them, and you, feel.

I have crossed paths with many such people in my walk of life and a few, in particular, in my local Kiwanis Club. These are not people you read about in the news. These are not even people who get awards because recognition is not their validator. Their validator is the goodness they know they are doing in their heart, like Cindy and her work with hospice. The angels among us.

One of my friends is such a woman. Her husband tragically died in a drag racing accident. I did not know her before, but I met her at our local Kiwanis Club. She wakes up each morning and starts doing for others: her son, her surrogate kids and grandkids, her neighbors, her friends, her community.

The problem is we don't hear these stories of people taking care of family or friends who just do for others. People who just grind. Who just keep doing good. The stories that are so abundant, but so underreported in our hard news world of "if it bleeds, it leads."

The people who just "do" don't need the affirmation of the outside world. They don't seek an award, recognition, or some sort of accolade. They simply do goodness because they want to. Because it is the gasoline in their motor of life. Because they know what is right. Because they know what makes them, and those they do their kindness for, feel good.

Please look. These people are everywhere, doing amazing acts, right there in your own community.

OUR START?

At Christmas time, my family and I have made it a point to join my Kiwanis Club and sing Christmas carols at convalescent homes. It is not much; it takes less than a few hours. We generally bring some friends, and my boys begrudgingly went along, for the first couple of years.

Then, something happened.

After Thanksgiving, the boys started asking, "When are we going to sing again?"

Now, I fully realize this is nothing earth-shattering by any stretch of the imagination, but perhaps this tiny bit of goodness, this "task" my wife and I would make them do, has now turned into something they look forward to.

There is so much goodness in this world. There is so much goodness happening right around the corner from you. My wish is that it become contagious within us all. Think of it. The power of compounding. We always hear about the power of compounding when speaking of money and savings and retirement: If I put this much away in my IRA and keep making those contributions in a 5 percent investment and never touch it, I will have this much when I retire. It is brilliant.

But "what if" we, collectively, made that same "investment" in making a difference in our communities and that compounded over time? That investment in goodness would grow just like the money in an IRA. And think about how much that would total if we all did it in our own small spheres of influence: whether within our own families, our communities, our nation. Think of the investment we would all have then.

It's not sexy, it's not flashy, and you may not get an award for it, or even a mention in your obituary, but just imagine. What would the exponential impact of this collective goodness be?

SELFLESS

My parents had some friends from church. My mom and Sue bonded quickly because of their German heritage and the fact that they both had three sons. We would go to each other's homes and enjoy barbecuing with our families. They had a baby girl ten years after their last son. The girl's name was Kim, and Sue and Steven asked my parents to be Kim's godparents.

Years later, Steven got transferred to Long Island for a new job. We would visit them, often taking a long car trip from Westchester to go to the beach for the day or stay overnight. Years later, Steven became sick and died of cancer. Sue moved closer to us and worked with my father. By now, Kim was starting high school. Then Sue became sick and, after a courageous battle with cancer, she too died.

Kim was fifteen and both her parents were gone. She immediately moved in with my parents and resumed her schooling. She instantly became part of our family, as her brothers were in different parts of the country trying to make their own ways. She fit right in.

How did Kim, at fifteen and having lost both her parents, find the strength to carry on?

I often think of the courage and strength of this woman, now my sister, and what she could have possibly felt at fifteen years of age with both her parents gone. How did she do it?

I also think of my parents' selfless act of love. As it so happened, my parents were empty nesters at the time and finally enjoying their time alone. Their three boys were off in various parts of the country starting their own lives. It was now their time, and they were young enough to enjoy their newfound freedom. But they also knew they had told Sue and Steven they would be Kim's godparents and that meant something to them.

You never think it is going to happen to you.

Sue is gone some thirty years at this time. Steven forty. Kim has lost a brother since then too. I know Kim has two blood brothers of her own, but Kim is my sister. She dug deep, and with the love and help of my parents, our family, her brothers, and many good friends, she has created a life of her own with two beautiful children and a loving husband. My parents made a difference in Kim's life and enriched our own in doing so. Their loving example has permeated through all of our lives.

IN SUM

The impact you have on this world does not have to be epic nor grand. There are many opportunities within your own community, your own neighborhood, your own family, that can be equally as impactful. What if we all, collectively, acted together on this small scale? Would the power of all those small acts compound the world over?

Start with your own family and watch that tiny ripple of hope build within your own pond. We teach selflessness by our actions in life. They are the actions that warrant no outward praise except from the ones closest to us. Together we can do this. I know we can do this together.

THE REMINDERS

Be a mentor to someone, however you define that.

There is so much goodness in the world already, just look.

Our impact does not have to be grand to make a difference.

Consider the exponential impact of collective goodness.

3 Avoid Judgment

He warned me. He warned me to be ready for this.

The door read "Staff only beyond this point."

I was now the owner. I was "staff."

I opened the door.

The white-hot fluorescent lights illuminated an already stark white room like only white-hot fluorescent lights can. The fetid smells of combined formaldehyde and human flesh permeated the thick air as the ancient wall unit struggled to pump freshness throughout the room. Two 1960s ceramic embalming tables lay side-by-side. The slight tilt in each enables "flow" down the drain.

On each table was a unique situation. Two posted bodies. (Posted simply means a coroner or specialist hired by the family is doing a postmortem evaluation of the body to determine a cause of death and perhaps its contributing factors. This happens when a family wants their own objective opinion of why their loved one died.) The scene does not look dissimilar from a *CSI* episode, a scary movie, or any other accurate depiction of this horrific but necessary part of death.

At this moment, it was as if time stopped for me. The scene was really quite surreal, perhaps best visualized to a layman as a kill site in the wild in which only the rib cage of a moose or other large animal has been left by the panoply of creatures who have previously fed off of it. But here, the layers of the dermis and epidermis hung off the table like slabs of meat, exposing these very human rib cages.

Combined with throat-gagging smells, the scene was horrifying. I was locked in the shock of seeing two posted bodies for the first time. These bodies were cut open, on full display, and were by far the most gruesome sight I had ever seen. As I stood there for a moment just looking at every internal part for the first time—a human spine, a liver, intestines—my eyes worked their way down the body and stopped on the two sets of feet: one white, one black. My pupils snapped back at the innards of these two exposed bodies lying side-by-side, then the feet, the innards, the feet.

A moment of complete clarity came over my thinking.

At that moment, the depiction of race in America, the stories of racism from around the globe, the xenophobia, the religious wars throughout the annals of human history of the world boiled down to this fluorescent-lit scene in an old funeral home's embalming room in Northern California.

I realized there is no difference among us humans at all. No difference in the inner composition of these two bodies to the human eye. True, we all have different colored and sized meat suits (our exteriors), and we all like different things; we are all unique. But, at our core, we are all the same—we human beings. What a complete and utter waste of time we all spend the world over attempting to delineate our differences.

Right here. Right now. In this very room was the picture we all need to see—two bodies of different race, splayed open, side-by-side—no difference on the inside.

I have seen it. No difference at all.

RACE, SEXUALITY, RELIGION, ETHNICITY, AND POLITICS

Nice, light topics, right? Now watch me lock this shit down in a few paragraphs.

I believe we live in an amazing country. A-ma-zing! It is a melting pot of many diverse and unique cultures, viewpoints, and people. In my opinion, that is what makes us truly unique. That, and the small fact that we are all allowed to speak our minds freely, according to the laws of our land.

'merica!

The problem arises when I try to convince you that I am right, and you are wrong. That my way is better than yours. That you need to understand my issues and me.

No, I don't.

I respect and acknowledge what, and who, you are. Just don't force your beliefs upon me. After all, I am unique. I think for myself. And I know I can join you, if I choose to. But it is my choice.

Again, America.

Look, God, or whoever you believe is running this show, is going to sort it all out in the end; don't take matters into your own hands and impose your beliefs on others; that's for someone far bigger than all of us. Nutshell. Mic drop. Peace out!

TONY

No one in the world taught me more about race in America than Tony Maynard.

As I mentioned earlier, I grew up going to Lutheran church every Sunday. We had a dynamic pastor named John Pearson. One of his passions was to bring inner-city kids out of New York City for the summer to live with the families of our church in and around Westchester County: towns like Pleasantville, Briarcliff Manor, and Armonk. He allied our church with Transfiguration Lutheran Church in Harlem, at the time a mostly African American community.

Each summer, boys and girls would be matched with families from our church, and the kids from their church would live with us for a few weeks. Insert your joke, anger, sarcasm, or ridicule here. But it was awesome and life-altering for me.

We had the same child for almost eight years, Tony Maynard. He was three years older than I, had a fro, used a pick to comb it, and had these naturally sleepy eyes and a wry smile. He was a little mischievous, an okay athlete, and he treated me like the little brother he never had. I thought he was literally the coolest guy on the face of the earth (like Dr. J times 100), and I remember looking forward to him coming every summer.

We generally did nothing too special when he came: went to friends' houses, played in the neighborhood, did a couple of church activities. I just loved having him around and how he watched out for me.

I vividly remember going to our public pool and playing Marco Polo. One day's game got particularly quiet as I had my eyes closed and called out to find my partner—

"Marco...?"

"MARCO...?"

"AHHH, MARCO... ?!!!!!!"

Then, the lifeguards' whistles blew like the warning sirens of Dresden and they pulled Tony off the bottom of the pool. After a precautionary night in the hospital, he was fine. (Mom said Tony hadn't gotten swimming lessons back home.)

Starting when he was fifteen, he came more infrequently. I remember the devastation hearing he was not coming that first summer because I looked so forward to seeing him.

My parents would hear from his mom. Periodically, he would make appearances at our house. My dad tried to instill in him a passion for civil engineering. Understandably, it did not take.

I heard he had gotten married. When I was working in the city one summer, I met Tony and his wife for dinner. He was the same guy: sleepy eyes, huge smile. Annie, his wife, was a kindred spirit from the day I met her. She loved her boys and she loved our Tony, warts and all.

More years and more distance went by. We heard stories from his mom of drug use and getting mixed up in "things." There would be years of hopefulness and getting straight. I always thought about him and remembered the summer days in Pleasant-ville, playing whiffle ball, eating ice cream from the Good Humor truck, a game of catch in the front yard, and sitting with him on the couch watching TV. I knew he loved me. I knew how he cared for me. He called me his brother.

The phone call came from my mother. Our Tony was dead. Tony had a heart attack on vacation with Annie and their boys.

When I was six years old, Tony Maynard taught me all I really ever needed to know about race, and, each year, his visits reinforced those beliefs. We were no different from one another. Sure, the color of our skin was different, but we really were no different from each other at all.

I know we will meet again. I truly do believe that. I have to. It gives me hope. It makes all this madness seem worthwhile. And we will laugh together like we used to—the silly, giddy, belly laughs of our youth. And in that better place, we will all smile, and we will love one another in a manner that is all too infrequent on this earth, but what Tony and I had here for a moment in time.

Until we meet again. Brothers forever.

IN SUM

The beauty of living in a democratic society is that certain rules and liberties are sacrosanct, and your voice can, and will, be heard. The bad part of living in a democratic society is that there are rules and liberties that are sacrosanct, and others' voices can, and will, be heard as well. We are entitled to speak our mind, even if those words may hurt someone.

For me, the Golden Rule is such a simple encapsulation of the way we should all go through life: "Do unto others as you would have them do unto you."

Terse, simple, perfect. No Higher Power would ever want you to take matters into your own hands to right the wrongs of society, no matter whom you believe in. I simply, inherently, believe this to be the ultimate truth.

And this is a great country in which to live. Compared to other parts of the world, the freedoms are unimaginable. We generally all want the same things: the best for our children and families, a chance to prosper, and freedom to be left alone to make decisions for ourselves. If we could all just do that and respect that in one another, I think we would be onto something. Spending time, and divisiveness, in delineating our differences furthers no true benefit in this world.

At our core, we are all the same.

THE REMINDERS

This is a great country.

Love is love, is love.

Please don't force me to be like you.

We are all the same, just different packaging.

---

4 Respect Others and Yourself

I was the last of our staff to arrive. Everyone was in place. The low-hanging fog was thick. It was the first funeral of the day in our local veterans' cemetery, one of the many hallowed final resting places for our country's veterans throughout the United States.

Rows and rows of white headstones stand at attention amid the dew-soaked grass. They head off into the dense fog as far as the foreboding day will let me see in this unbelievably austere setting. Each stone marks the spot of a veteran (and maybe their spouse) who gave everything for our country.

You simply cannot set foot on this soil without feeling respect, without feeling honor, without feeling pride and dignity.

At the gravesite, a casket draped with Old Glory was perched majestically above its final resting place on the hunter green straps of the casket lift above the dug out soil of the grave.

The sound rose softly in the distance as the bugles played "Taps." It is as impactful a moment as I have felt. Its sounds crippling the already serene setting with its haunting, yet triumphant sound bellowing through the early day's air.

To hear this music, in this setting, is respect personified.

As the buglers finished, we heard the command, "Present arms!"

A few soldiers raised guns to the sky in perfect unison.

The shots sounded like an explosion…and then twenty more in succession.

The widow and her daughter gripped each other's hands tighter, their white knuckles visible from my distance.

When the last gun fired, the echo of its blast lingered forever in this former desolate farmland.

Shortly after, two soldiers marched up to the casket. Like a choreographed ballet, they carefully and respectfully lifted the American flag off the casket. They folded it slowly, methodically, first, in half, then again, one more time. One pulled it tight as the other gripped even tighter with their white-gloved hands. No creases here. Then, one soldier slowly folded a corner, then another, toward his compatriot, creating constant small, taut triangles, one after the other. Eventually, he was right in front of the other soldier. He folded it even tighter and tucked the remaining piece of cloth into a crevice created by the fabric; Old Glory was now folded in triangular perfection.

It is awesome to witness the ceremony of the flag folding: two men of precision, our country's flag, perfect sync.

When they were complete, one soldier handed the triangular package to the other soldier. He marched slowly, methodically, respectfully to the widow, got down on one knee, and expressed the thanks "from a grateful nation" for her family's sacrifice. He handed her the flag and marched back to join his fellow soldier.

The whole ceremony takes less than ten minutes, but it should be witnessed by everyone in our nation. This is respect personified and a must-see once in your lifetime, much like the changing of the guard at the Tomb of the Unknown Solider at Arlington Cemetery in Washington.

Thank you for your service.

MR. GOODWIN

My Opa (German for grandfather) came to America on a boat, not speaking a word of English. His father sent him in exchange for money his brother lent their family back in Germany to keep their family sawmill business afloat. As Opa worked the streets of New York City delivering milk, eggs, and cheese to delis and luncheonettes, he saved every penny so he could afford to bring his new bride (back in Germany) to America.

After a few months in the New World, he did just that. And my grandparents kept it going, continuing to save each and every penny, to better their lives. Probably like many of our immigrant grandparents, he worked every day: day in, day out, nose down, grinding.

When he saved up a little cash, he asked his uncle what he should do with his extra money. His uncle John introduced him to his attorney, Leo Goodwin, who advised my grandfather how to invest his hard-earned savings. Now, I am quite certain, Mr. Goodwin had any number of opportunities over his lifetime to do the wrong thing and take this money from an unsuspecting immigrant and either steal it or place him in some risky, pie-in-the-sky investment.

But he never did that.

Instead, he invested my grandfather's money in solid blue-chip stocks starting in and around the mid-1930s.

My grandfather never questioned him, he just kept handing over more and more money as he saved it, watching every stock split two for one, every dividend reinvestment, his money compounding annually. Simple investing.

Why did Mr. Goodwin do this? Why did Mr. Goodwin not take advantage of a situation that would have been like taking candy from a baby? Why was this man so good?

Mr. Goodwin's advice paid off. My grandfather was a millionaire when he retired at the age of sixty-five. A man who delivered milk, eggs, and cheese up and down the streets of New York City was a millionaire by the time he retired.

If that is not the American Dream, then what is?

I will never forget Leo Goodwin's name as long as I live. Honor, respect, trust: the basis of the way we should all live and treat one another.

And my grandfather…he didn't stop there.

He could have traveled the world over to wonderful ports of call, spent lavishly on the so-called finer things, indulged on anything and everything he worked so hard for all those endless days and nights in an un–air-conditioned truck on the hot, asphalt streets of New York City.

But that was not him.

Instead, he told my parents he wanted to pay for his grandsons' educations. My grandfather sent the three of us to college and paid half of the tuition for two law schools—this at a time when my father was at the critical juncture of starting his own business out of our home and every penny mattered. It enabled my father to take bigger risks than he would have, if he had three college educations to pay for. And my father would be the first to tell you that.

You see, for my grandfather, it was about his family.

Early on in their marriage my grandparents made a pact to always "help the boys" (we three grandsons). Since his wife had predeceased him, paying for our education was his way of honoring the pact he made with his wife, paying homage to her in a way that was much more fulfilling than anything else he could spend his money on.

This immigrant with a sixth-grade education wanted nothing more than for his three grandsons to have more education than he had—way more.

He affected so many different lives with that decision. My dad could expand his business with the extra money; my mom could stay home and help him; and we three did not have the albatross of college debt.

What if we all did unselfish acts like this in our lifetimes? Fantastic things!

What if we all just said I am going to invest in my family instead of spending my money on the material trappings of society that advertising execs the world over make us think we need?

What if? No, seriously, what if?

SOMETIMES RESPECT WORKS AGAINST YOU

After I made a low-budget movie in New York City in the early 1990s and it didn't get into the Sundance Film Festival, I was crestfallen. I talked with my mom about what my future held. I expressed an interest in working for my father's business, a thriving consulting firm of forty people, with the hope of maybe taking it over one day.

My father said, "No."

He said I had no experience and he wasn't sure I could bring any value to the firm. (I was a licensed New York State attorney with a master's in environmental law at the time.)

I never spoke directly to my father about it because it came through his interpreter. My mom explained, "Your father doesn't feel it would be fair to the men and women who have worked so hard with him for all these years."

Respect.

He was mindful of the entitled son taking over a business in which he had no experience. Harsh.

If you were me, yes. But I suspect it was an easy decision for my father.

Years later my father was ready to retire and sold the business to a few of his coworkers. His lifelong accountant told him he was giving the business away by doing the deal. My father didn't care. He realized if he got fair market value for his company, his coworkers would have been too cash-strapped to survive. He saw that exact scenario with his former employer, some twenty years prior, and he thought it was greedy of his former boss to do that to his colleagues.

I moved to California and I returned for the holidays and every summer to visit. Still do. Does my dad think what might have been if he had let his son take over his company? My life would have been very different. His life would have been very different.

Looking back on it now, I have no bitterness. It challenged me to grow as a man, to try things I am certain I would have never had the courage to do, like write a book.

My father respected his work family above his own flesh and blood. I think, next to marrying my mom, not hiring me was the best decision of his life.

YOURSELF

This story is a perfect segue into respecting yourself. For me, it was the harsh reality of looking in the mirror and realizing there was no easy way out. I know this is difficult for most of us to do and that is why I want to talk about it because looking in the mirror, figuratively and literally, is the best thing we can do when we are struggling.

Whether it is a rough family situation, popping Oxys like they're cherry Skittles, a bad business decision, trying to discover if you can see through the empty bottle of Smirnoff, picking up your clothes from another encounter you mistakenly got yourself into, chasing the dragon, or a relationship that simply will not work, we have all been there. We have all been there. All of us. It's called being human. Your failures, no matter how grave, are the foundation.

You are worth another chance: If not from family, if not friends, if not clergy, if not a social worker, there are plenty of people in the world who still want to help.

You are worth it. I know it. I know it with every fiber of my soul. Believe it!

IN SUM

I believe in the days of yesteryear when respect meant something. Born from the type of men my father and grandfather are/were, men of a seemingly bygone era. I want that era back. We need that era back in America. Sure, sometimes it works against you, but the lessons learned, no matter how harsh, will last a lifetime. And, hopefully, the lessons learned will change the person you become to pass on to another generation of family members.

I understand times are changing and the world is rapidly evolving around us, but when did respect lose its sexiness? What if we all treated each other with more respect, if corporations practiced the same to its shareholders, if sons and daughters understand, like me, that opportunities are not just given because of your bloodlines? If we all understood that hard work should be canonized, whatever vocation that might be, only then I think we would have something as a society.

Respect.

THE REMINDERS

We need to get back to respecting one another.

Corporations need to learn respect too.

True respect teaches us reality.

Respecting ourselves is the first step.

Alcoholics Resource Center: (800) 839-1686
(https://alcoholicsanonymous.com)

Substance Abuse and Mental Health Services
Administration: (800) 662-4357 (https://www.
samhsa.gov/find-help/national-helpline)

5　Be Vulnerable

A young man died. His family came in to make arrangements; there were a lot of family members in that room. It was a rougher crowd: leather vests, jeans, motorcycle boots, ink aplenty.

The child's mother was naturally wrecked. Destroyed. The dad cooler, stoic, emotionless.

After they had decided what they wanted, they asked me if they could make payments. I explained that our funeral home did not do that. We refused to perform any services prior to having them paid for.

I explained they could opt for a cremation and how that was significantly cheaper.

This was an affront to them. "There is no way you're gonna burn my son."

Nice job, Chris. I thought to myself.

We sat there in awkward silence.

The mother broke into tears, again. A couple of men in the room just stared at me. Not like blank stares, more like stares you get late at night in a bar when you look at a guy's girlfriend a little too long.

But I stuck to my guns. I had to. It's the funeral "business," right?

They left and said they would return with the money. I was not optimistic.

A few hours later, I got a call from our local cemetery. The manager asked, "Chris, you gonna do that funeral?"

I explained I would, if I got paid. He told me they had no money, and he told them he could not bury their son without being paid first either. I told my cemetery compatriot I totally understood and that we had told the family the same thing. It is the unfortunate part of our business.

Both the burial and funeral were scheduled for a week later.

As the days passed, I held the spot open for the family to have the service. Much to my surprise, the family came in two hours before the scheduled service and handed me $7,000 in cash. We agreed to perform the service. I will not lie when I tell you I went into the back office and ran a Dri Mark pen over every bill to make sure they weren't counterfeit. I am not that noble.

The cemetery called me and reiterated that they had not been paid, and they would not bury according to the family's wishes. They simply would not. No matter how many people showed up. I told them I understood and that I would inform the family.

When I told the family, they said a friend was bringing the money shortly.

We performed the memorial service at our funeral home. It was packed as it usually is when a young person dies. There was no room in the parking lot, no extra seats in the chapel; in fact, we were overflowing to the outside of the funeral home.

It was a moving service in which friends, brothers and sisters, and family spoke of their love for this young man. You start to identify with people when you listen to their stories.

When the service ended, everyone was just milling about asking questions about the funeral procession to the cemetery. I could see the family talking. The mother and father slowly walked over to me and asked if we could talk in my office.

When we got there, the mother erupted in tears, shouting how she cannot bury her baby boy and went into hysterics. The father calmly explained that the friend had not been able to raise the money for the cemetery.

I sat there looking at this woman crying for her son, slumped over in my office. The crowd was growing outside my office door as the mourners had now seeped into the foyer and were peeking in at the wailing woman. And the numbers were swelling.

I could feel my conscience asking what if this were my son—as the bulge of greenbacks pressed against my leg, protruding from my suit pant pocket as only a thick wad of bills can. I could feel my vulnerability coursing through my mind.

You're an asshole if you don't let this woman bury her son. You'll go out of business if you're this vulnerable with every grieving family in this situation. What do I do?

I reached into my pocket, pulled out their $7,000 in cash, and handed it to the mother. "Go bury your son."

She stopped crying, rose too quickly, and said, "We'll pay you back next week," and, WHOOSH, they were out the door.

Dang.

They buried their son. I saw them. My cemetery buddy came

over to me, and out of the corner of his mouth said, "Not in a million years did I think they'd ever come up with that money."

I turned to him and smiled. He kept looking at me. "You got paid, Chris, right?"

I looked back at the crowd at the grave.

"Chris?"

I was vulnerable that day and I got taken. It stung. We were just starting out in business, and I had that seven grand in my hand. I was vulnerable and I got played.

Never let that dissuade you. The sting subsides and this is your human connection to the world.

Kindness over money…any day.

A FRIEND OF BILL

One of the greatest displays of vulnerability I have witnessed was a college girlfriend, the first true love of my life.

Katy and I had been dating a couple of years when she took me aside one day and said she had a problem. I was in my early twenties, so millions of thoughts exploded through my mind like fireworks: She's preggers, found another dude, doesn't like my Drakkar Noir. I was truly scared.

Then she said it. "I have a drinking problem."

"What do you mean?" I asked.

"I have a drinking problem: I drink, I black out, I don't remember what happened the night before."

"Come on, I do the same thing," I chided.

"No, you know when to stop. I don't."

"Pleeeeeeeese," I said.

More stares. But now I saw she was completely serious.

A beat.

"I wanna go to AA."

Alcoholics Anonymous? I shouted to no one but myself inside my own head with eyes widened.

"I want you to take me."

But how could this be? We're from nice families, I thought to myself. We live in nice houses. You have a pool. Our dads are successful. Our moms are in the PTA. Ya know, the rational, mature kinds of things a twenty-year-old mind thinks.

But she wasn't playing. Simply looking into her eyes, I knew. A long beat and I said, "Of course, I'll take you."

I pulled her close for a long embrace as a million more thoughts fired through my young brain: She's not an alcoholic, she's just sad. What does this mean for me? How can we ever party again? Maybe it's just temporary. I'll go to make her feel better. I don't like Perrier. What if someone sees me at the meeting? What will my parents think? Do her parents know? There is no way I—

"Thank you," she replied as she pulled back and looked deeper into my eyes. "I thought you would freak out."

"Me?"

I hear she is nearing thirty years sober. I had nothing to do with her success in the program. I think about her courage and vulnerability at that moment all these years removed from that day. I admire what that must have taken, in that particular moment, at such a young age.

Vulnerability is an amazing thing.

MY YOUNGER SELF?

It is the first day of high school for my incoming freshman son.

The car was deafeningly quiet, as only it can be with a fourteen-year-old surfing on his phone; only the sounds of the car motor are humming as we drove to school. Then I noticed the look on his face.

"You nervous?"

"Yeah," he immediately responded, which he never does when locked onto his phone.

"'Bout what?"

A long beat of staring at the car's floorboards.

"Gonna be weird, ya know, showering."

Wow.

"It was weird for me too," I quickly added.

"Not super excited about it."

"I wasn't either. Some kids are more mature and guys like us, not so much. I was the same as you," trying desperately to show our common bond.

He looked into my eyes. I saw fear. Real fear. In that instant, I recollected the same fear I had forty years earlier. It was déjà vu all over again.

Eyes back to his phone.

A long beat.

"You gotta do it. It'll be even weirder if you're that kid that never showers."

He nodded as my car pulled to a stop at school.

He opened the door. He was scared. Really scared.

"You got this."

He nodded and sloughed off.

I would say this was one of the most vulnerable moments of my son's life thus far. And he trusted me enough to share his fears. I didn't lie. I was there too. I remember that day like it was this morning, football in ninth grade, my first shower with the team, and I wasn't as mature as most guys.

Will they tell all the girls in class tomorrow? Will everyone know my secret? How will I ever be able to walk the hallways again? Will everyone stare at me? Will no one take me seriously because I am not as mature as most other guys?

An absolutely crushing part of growing up. You really see where you stand at fourteen, and you can't possibly comprehend that things will even out in just a year or two.

The seminal moment of adolescence.

I was grateful my son chose to share his fears with me. Talk about vulnerability.

IN SUM

Vulnerability is difficult because if you get burned even once, you tend to withdraw from that hurt for a long time. But don't. Don't, because the person who let you down is the one with the problem. You just got your answer way faster than investing any more time in them—victory, not defeat. And, when you have vulnerability in a relationship, you truly have something. The person you have been with has shown their mettle. It gets good after this.

Don't be afraid. Let your guard down. It tells you so much more about people than if you would never have let it down in the first place.

THE REMINDERS

Be vulnerable to those you trust; if they don't support you, you do not want them in your life.

In terms of family, always be vulnerable.

Share your stories with your children. It will bond you.

---

6 Get Uncomfortable

When I started in the funeral industry, I felt I had to do and see it all, if I was going to expect the same of my coworkers. I was, however, not particularly excited about picking up decedents from the coroner's office initially, and forever more for that matter.

The coroner's office is where decedents go when anything funky happens or there is no next of kin. They determine why someone died, to make sure there was no criminal act. If there was a criminal act, the coroner assists the police in their investigation to determine who is responsible. You've watched *Bones*.

This is where you see things you can't unsee: bodies found after long periods of time, bodies found in water, burned victims, traffic accidents—you name it.

In my opinion, coroner employees are unbelievable human beings because this is their job and they chose it.

Mad respect.

I remember going to the coroner early in my career as a funeral guy to pick up a decedent and bring them back to the funeral home.

You back your van up, take your collapsible Ferno cot out of the back, wheel it in, and fill out your paperwork.

Usually, a supremely overworked individual will take your cot and go to the coroner's industrial cooler to remove the body. In larger, more metropolitan jurisdictions, you are generally not allowed past a certain point, which was totally fine with me.

I would generally stare at the ceiling and think about how my degrees were really coming in handy about now, and how proud my parents must be.

The pick-up process was generally the same: Make sure the name the coroner had on the decedent's wrist or ankle matched the one you were about to place on their ankle, load up the family's loved one, strap them in for the ride, and drive off.

On this particular trip to a small, remote jurisdiction, it was different. They had very specific times in which you could pick up because they were drastically understaffed. In this coroner's office in a quasi-public county set of buildings, I rang a doorbell as you would at your neighbor's home.

A man in a smock answered the door and I said, "I'm here for a pick up."

He let me in, and we filled out the paperwork.

"Did they tell you about this?"

"What?"

"He's a jumper."

"A what?"

"A jumper. He jumped off the bridge and was found in the gorge."

"Yeah, no, they forgot those details."

"There's not much here. I am gonna need some help."

"Help?"

"Like picking him up."

"I thought I wasn't supposed to go past that line?" turning and praying to find that same line in the cement as the city coroner's office.

Nope.

I slowly turned back around as he was saying, "You see anyone else who can help me?"

He laughed and already had the door to the cooler open. The cooler was the kind with the sliding drawers, just like you see on TV or in the movies. He slid the seven-foot stainless steel tray out. On the stainless tray was a body bag. (There are two kinds of body bags: regular and industrial strength.)

This was industrial strength.

I reached for the zipper to place the ID tag on the decedent's ankle as was always the first step in every removal I did.

"You don't want to do that," the coroner said.

"Sorry, it's our company protocol," I naively said.

"No!" he forcefully replied as he reached into a drawer behind him and pulled out packing tape.

"Put your ID tag on the bag."

"No, I—"

"Do it!"

I followed his orders and he taped the ID tag to the bag.

"Now give me a hand." He slid my cot over to the body and instructed me where to grab. We picked up the bag and it felt like picking up a water bed.

We placed him on the cot, and I quickly extracted my arms.

I looked back at the coroner.

I now fully understood why we taped the ID to the outside of the bag. The coroner knew what was inside. He saw I was new at this. He was watching out for me.

I headed back to the funeral home in my van and tried to shake the feel of that body bag from my mind. As my thoughts selfishly focused on me and what I was feeling, my conscience decided to take a right turn and remind me of the parts of the boy lying in a body bag in the rear of my van.

What about his discomfort? What was he thinking at that critical moment in his life? Why?

My front seat feelings suddenly took a backseat wishing I could have helped him in his time of need. There are so many souls out there who need us. Our kind words, our words of encouragement, our help.

I tried to shake the thoughts of him from my mind. I literally shook my head to free them.

But I can't. They are here forever. The indelible mark of discomfort that forms the appreciation for something greater, something way greater.

IN THE BEGINNING

I wrote what I thought was the most beautiful letter to my eldest son upon his graduation from eighth grade. I poured out my heart to share the story of how he came to be.

It was a legendary letter of love.

I placed it next to his bed conspicuous enough for a blind man to see.

My fourteen-year-old son never even acknowledged that I

wrote it. Weeks later, when I asked him if he read it, he said, "It was long."

Long.

He was way more enamored with his friend's parents who gave their son $3,000 to buy whatever he wanted.

Anyway, that's not why I wrote it.

I wrote my son that letter to share with him a history of us. I wrote him a letter of how he, his mother, and I became a family. I wanted to tell him about a time in my life when I was extremely uncomfortable, in a pickle really.

When he was born, we had nothing. I was an unemployed screenwriter in Hollywood, and his mom was working as a PR executive making all of our money. Holding that child in my arms, with no regular job, and his wondrous blues looking up at me was like a Tyson right-handed, uppercut to my unsuspecting genitals.

Life-altering doesn't seem to capture the gravity of that child's look.

Angie and I brought him home from Cedars-Sinai Medical Center and just stared at him. Then at each other. Then him. Then each other.

Life just got really real. In that one fleeting moment, no words were exchanged, but everything was said.

What do we do now? we thought in sync.

I remember Angie's eyes as we looked at each other. It's one thing when the kid's in the belly, but this…

Neither of us knew a thing, not a freakin' thing. Sure, we had read all the books (*What to Expect When You're Expecting* by Heidi Murkoff was our personal bible), but this…

We gave him his first bath, put too much soap on him, and had our own built-in, porcelain Slip 'N Slide. He was like an oversized, stuffed turkey rolling around our bathtub; I swear we should've had a helmet on him. My mother-in-law was bellied over laughing, literally bellied over, watching our ineptitude. I know she told that story to many friends.

So I explained all this to Hud. How my life changed when we had him.

Thirty-nine years of age. Unemployed. Newborn. No viable job or prospects on the horizon. Wife who wants to be a mom.

What the hell had I gotten us into?

I had been out of the law field for too long to go back and start a career, especially if I wanted to see him at night and have more children.

A friend of my wife's family (a mortician) had been encouraging me to start a funeral home with him. He said it was a secure industry (people always die) and he knew the ropes.

After discussing options with my wife, I found out she wanted to raise our family near her family in Northern California. There weren't exactly any opportunities jumping out at me back East, so, as it turned out, a funeral home, of all possibilities, was my best option.

Insert your joke here.

It was not comfortable. It was not what I always dreamed of. It was not my passion or lifelong desire to take care of the grieving and the lost. But I was motivated by this child's beautiful azure, blue circles looking up at me, as if saying, "Take care of me. Help me. Show me what all this is."

So I kissed him and my wife and left for a city I had never been to before. Me, the homebody, who wanted to be a writer, hit the road. I went to Northern California to scout potential locations for a new funeral home.

I would scout locations around the city all day and sleep on my friend's couch at night. I stayed there so often I told him and his roommate I would pay half the rent. I would head back home on weekends to see my wife and son and head back to scout locations week after week. Then, one day, we heard a local funeral home was having financial troubles.

Did I "will" this to happen? Did I put good juju out into the universe to make this happen?

We purchased the funeral business with the help of my parents and turned the place around, restoring it to its former grace. I knew nothing about the funeral industry, only the obvious, to treat people with dignity and respect. It was baptism by fire.

Our mortician friend always asked me if I was sure I wanted to take the next step behind the curtain. I always said yes. I had to; I had a new child and wife to care for. No matter how uncomfortable, I had to learn.

In my eyes, there is no greater time to grow and become strong than when you have no other option—the last resort. My newborn son did that for me.

We found a house, moved in, and started to make it our home: me at work and Angie taking care of Hud. The greatest luxury I had was coming home and seeing their smiling faces.

It was all the motivation I needed.

So, in my opinion, getting uncomfortable is when good things happen. It tests you; it shows what you are made of in a way it never will when you are comfortable and contented.

When you're uncomfortable, good things happen.

COLLEGE

I had a similar period of discomfort in college. In my mind I was way smarter than my grades (or SAT scores) indicated. I had clearly not "applied" myself in high school. (How many times have I heard that phrase from a parent? I just love it.) Anyway, "application" did not happen in high school for me, but I thought of myself as smart.

I was delusional.

I thought I should be going to Boston College or Tufts. As it turned out, the Boston College and Tufts admissions' offices thought I was delusional too.

I got into a few schools, but chose Purdue University in West Lafayette, Indiana, not really knowing anything about Purdue University in West Lafayette, Indiana.

I remember rolling up I-65 North with my mom. As we drove, I looked left. Right. I looked forward. Back. Flat. Real flat. The kid who had spent the first eighteen years of his life in the wooded properties of Westchester County, New York, was in full-blown culture shock.

I still remember my mother pulling away from my dorm on the far northwest side of campus and me thinking, what in God's name have I gotten myself into?

I thought about tearing off down the street after my mom's now disappearing red Subaru before snapping out of that cold sweat only to realize my three roommates were staring at me clearly thinking, yeah, we know you wanna run after Mommy... ya lil' bitch.

So that began an extremely uncomfortable period in my life. My sole mission from that day forward was to get in the library, get good grades, and transfer back East. Immediately! I soon found out the schools did not accept students until the middle of their sophomore years.

I had, at least, a year and a half there.

So I worked. I really worked.

I was in the stacks every night, even on Fridays, studying. When the grades came in the mail (I know, I am old), I remember opening the letter and seeing how well I had done. I actually dropped to my knees and started crying. I had never wanted something so badly in all my life.

It was probably the first time I had challenged myself academically, and it paid off. I was uncomfortable out there, and I wanted to go to school near my brother in Boston. I worked my tail off and it paid off. I transferred to Brandeis University (just outside Boston), and I lived with my brother. We had some magical years there together.

IN SUM

If you are reading this and have doubt, let me guarantee you this. Any time you really want something, it is attainable, no matter how fantastic. But you gotta put in the legit work. Sometimes it only takes a semester. Sometimes it takes a year. Sometimes many years. But if you are true to yourself, and the task at hand, it eventually works.

The great part about being in a bad situation, or at the bottom of anything, is that there is only one way to go. The problem people have with being uncomfortable, in my opinion, is that they get stuck and dwell in that discomfort. That is to say, your discomfort will not stop unless you do something to get yourself out of said discomfort. And since there is only one way to go, I see that as a pretty good cost-benefit. Do something to get out of your bad situation, do not dwell in it!

THE REMINDERS

From the soil of discomfort sprout the seeds of greatness.

Work. Work every day toward a goal and it will be attained.

Uncomfortable is a great starting place for something big.

---

7 Failure Is the Foundation

It was kind of an ordinary day. The day you kind of just go along for the ride. You don't think too much about the larger life issues. Just get through the nine-to-five, finish all your work, and get home to the family.

I was sitting in the back of the chapel at this memorial service. I do this if I am running the service to make sure I am present when the time is right to get people to the cemetery for their final stop, literally and figuratively.

Then the words of the speaker started resonating.

He was speaking about his father. He was doing what most people do, in sharing with the attendees, his audience today, an abridged version of his father's life—a necessary but evil tradition in funerals, in my opinion, because how do you tell about your father's (or mother's, brother's, or anyone's) life, all the things they did, in a palatably timed speech to keep your audience's attention?

You can't.

But it's expected.

It seems his dad was a tinkerer. He tinkered in his shop. He tinkered with all kinds of experiments: some wood, some electronics, some gadgets.

So this son started picking up the speed of his speech. He was clearly hummin' now in his syncopation and delivery. Most noticeable was the word that ended each little story, in tones that appeared to be getting louder and louder—

Failure.

Failure!

FAILURE!

As the pace of his eulogy increased, it started to get a little uncomfortable. There was rustling in the chapel rows too. If you've been to a few of these, you can see it from a mile away—or at least from the back row. It is clear some in attendance felt what I was feeling.

But the son's pace and dogmatic oratory did not stop.

Now I was glued to this speaker as if listening to Abraham Lincoln deliver a proclamation. Or witnessing an implosion. Like I have seen many times at funerals in which the speaker is so overcome with emotion that they can no longer hold it together and they shatter in a fiery human explosion at the pulpit before an audience of family and friends.

The train wreck you can't look away from.

No, this man, this son, was right on a razor's edge, like the ultrafine gut of a Stradivarius string. But then he suddenly stopped, sweat now pouring off him. He stared into the crowd, panting. We all were hanging on his next words.

Silence.

Will he speak?

Did we all just witness a son's breakdown?

"My dad was anything but a failure. Society may have thought he failed because a business didn't work, or an idea didn't, or a prototype never made it to the patent office, but my father...my god, my father instilled in me and my sisters that anything, anything in life was possible. And his tinkering, his daily, his weekly, his yearly tinkering, simply confirmed that too.

"He didn't care what society told him. He was just sharing with his kids. He showed me and my sisters what he loved. What he thought about in his head. What he thought might be possible.

"A failure?

"No, he showed us how failures, how his failures, our failures, bore the seeds of critical thinking that make dreams and ideas possible."

Silence. Heads nodded in total silence.

Daaaaaamn!

I was blown away in the backseat of a chapel that day—no ordinary day.

MEL

When I was in Hollywood trying to be a screenwriter, I was extremely dedicated to the craft, regularly writing for eight to ten hours a day. To be able to do this, I got seasonal work from November through January running the Academy Award campaign for Paramount Classics, the art house division of Paramount Pictures.

It was a great education of how Hollywood movies attempted to get nominated for an Academy Award. I would send screeners out (DVD or CDs) to each member of the Academy so they could watch each film being nominated for consideration in the comfort of their home and, hopefully, vote for our studio's films. When I worked there, we had Sofia Coppola's *The Virgin Suicides* and Ken Lonergan's *You Can Count on Me*, which was nominated for Best Original Screenplay. This was an unexpected coup for such a small art house division of a major studio—due to nothing I did.

It was amazing how many films went out to all the members of the Academy, over 5,800 people receiving every movie each studio was pushing for Academy Award consideration each year. This is a whole subculture of the movie industry few people know about.

I was good at my job and really liked the people I worked with. The head of my division, Ruth Vitale, was one of the first women of the art house movie scene. She had a great eye for finding such films and was well thought of in the industry. She was also tough, truly the prototypical LA power broker straight out of a caricature film like *Get Shorty*, although her denizens were simply the art house world of cinema. She could be rough on coworkers, and she liked to be escorted in from her car on a daily basis. When she was arriving, the entire office knew.

It was a high pucker moment each and every day.

"Duck, Ruth is coming" could be heard whispered through the second-floor hallways.

She, sort of, liked me (tolerated me, really) because I think she respected that I had made a film of my own, and she knew how difficult that was. She knew I was capable of much more, so she recommended me when Mel Gibson was looking for an assistant.

That's how I came to sit down with Mel—just Mel Gibson and me.

Now mind you, he had already won an Academy Award for directing and acting in *Braveheart*, and he had already made *The Patriot* (which I called "American Revolution Braveheart" to no one but myself), and he was the highest paid actor/producer in Hollywood at the time, truly at the top of his game.

I, being the ambitious, aspiring screenwriter trying to make an impression, got ahold of his next script, *We Were Soldiers*, written by none other than Academy Award–winning writer of *Braveheart*, Randall Wallace. Weeks before the interview, right up until the very night before the interview, I read and reread that script from all possible angles.

I knew that script better than Mr. Wallace did.

I went to the interview in one of these lovely offices on the Paramount lot off Gower. I was greeted by one of Mel's producing partners who walked me into the garden area and made small talk, probably to make sure I wasn't crazy, didn't smell of Camembert, and wasn't carrying any concealed weaponry.

I sat for a couple of minutes when the door opened and out walked Mel. He was wearing a flannel shirt, blue jeans, and casual shoes, that may have even been Birkenstocks. I am 6 feet 2, so he appeared small to me, and he had that shifty eye *Lethal Weapon*–type presence that made you feel as if he could go off at any moment. He appeared steely and reserved, definitely not a hugger.

I had done my homework and knew he was born near where I grew up in New York. He didn't seem to be too impressed with that.

So much for the small talk.

We talked briefly about the job and what it would entail, and it seemed like I could handle it pretty easily. He explained he was about to shoot his new movie *We Were Soldiers* ("Vietnam Braveheart," I thought to myself) and asked if I had read it.

"Well, hells yeah," I shouted in my mind only.

Now was my time.

I could feel it. You could feel it. Heck, the greater cosmos could feel it.

You see, I was never that star-adoring sycophant that most Hollywood assistants were. I didn't want to be "that" guy, that "yes" man, that idol worshipper. I was my own man, and I wanted to show Mel that, ya know, because he would respect that; this was the guy who made *Braveheart*, for god's sake, one of my favorite movies of all time.

At that moment, at that very moment, I felt as if my face was painted blue and I was rushin' down the fens right next to Mel with a frickin' pickaxe in my hand about to hurl that semi-glistening piece of rust 'n blood–encrusted metal into some unsuspecting Englishman's neck.

I was gonna slay that script!

I quickly snapped out of it and proceeded to tell Mel the story had problems (ya know, the story Academy Award–winning screenwriter Randall Wallace wrote) because it lacked a love interest for the main character and that felt very uneven to me.

I saw his crystal blue eyes shoot over to my now fawning hazels.

Really? I knew he was thinking.

I may have soiled myself in that very instance, but for some reason the voice in my larynx ignored my briefs and just kept going as if on Tesla autopilot.

I then went on a well-documented, ten-minute diatribe about the lack of a love interest and how audiences need, nay, expect, that from these types of Hollywood movies, because I am such a pro, the unemployed screenwriter, living in a shed—

DOWN BY THE FRICKIN' RIVER!

And as God is my witness, Mel sat there and listened. He listened to every word I had to say and never interrupted. Not once.

And when I had finished, he looked over at me and paused. Like a long, frickin' pause.

I felt the Eggo duo I had for breakfast rising in my throat.

Then Mel asked me if I had ever gotten into a fight?

I looked up at him for a beat and our eyes met. Goddamn, they were a pretty blue.

And in that very moment, I thought…

Is Mel Gibson gonna lay me out?

Is Mel Gibson gonna come flying off the top turnbuckle and fire a throat punch to my juice hole in this serene garden-like setting off Gower on the Paramount lot?

I said yes that I had gotten the tar beaten out of me after mouthing off to a gang of guys at college while in a state of extreme inebriation. That seemed to make sense to Mel.

In retrospect, I believe his small homily to me that day was his kind way of saying, "Get the hell out of my sight and make sure I never see you again in my eyesight as long as I, or you, are in Hollywood."

As it turns out, my tenure was much shorter than his.

When I returned to work the next week, Ruth, the head of our studio, asked me into her office. She sat me down and asked, "What the hell happened?"

I told her the whole story and of my rationale for dissecting the script and the problems it had, almost verbatim, as I had explained to Mel during the interview. She just looked at me for what seemed like an eternity, mouth agape. (She was an attractive woman rockin' a fresh coiffed bob.)

But now it started to get uncomfortable.

I gave her that look like…

What?

And she said, "You idiot."

I deserved that.

"You FUCKIN' idiot!"

She was Catholic, so she held back.

"You thought it was a good idea to dissect an Academy Award–winning writer's script to an Academy Award–winning actor, director, and producer?"

See, in hindsight, when she said laid it all out as clearly as that, I should have said no, but I said, "Ya…es?"

And just like that her assistant, Joe, opened the door, looked right at me, and smiled, and I knew which direction I should go. Straight to hell!

So when you hear all of those people like me saying, "Fail, fail, failure is good, it teaches you so much." Just sit back in your chair, smile, and remember my story because whatever you just failed at probably wasn't as legendary a failure as mine.

The thing that is tough about failure is that when it happens to you, you feel so alone, so singularly all alone in that moment that it exacerbates the already bad feelings (of failure) you have and forces you to spiral and overthink the situation, causing even more heightened feelings of failure. While self-reflection and thinking about your failure is good, it is never really as bad as it feels in the moment.

Case in point, when I walked out of Ruth's office that day, I felt like crap. That feeling only grew by the next day when I was fairly certain the entire office had heard of my failure. As I walked the halls, (whether real or not) in my mind I thought there were stares, whispers, snickers, and idle glances from the usual suspects. And to make matters worse, I was "the part-time guy," only brought in to do a few months' job, already an outsider in this overly cliquey workplace. I rationalized back and forth in my mind that no one knew anything, then everyone knew, then no one, then everyone, ultimately convincing myself that my story was safe.

Until one of my coworkers stormed up to me, pulled me aside, and whispered to me like he was selling trade secrets to the North Koreans: "Did it really happen?"

"What?"

"Did you really rip Mel's script to shit right in front of his face?"

"No, I would never—"

"You're a frickin' god," and he quickly scampered off before anyone else would see me with him.

Your failures are your own. They are unique to you. They are special. Put the blinders on and keep trying; you never know how they are perceived to others.

IN SUM

People of the world, trust your gut. It is the greatest barometer of right and wrong you have: You must fail to succeed, you must be embarrassed to become confident, and you must hurt to love. Look at failure as a building block to your success; if you never take that first step, you are paralyzed—safe, but paralyzed—and you will not have lived.

With each failure, learn something new and do not make the same mistake again. If you do keep making the same mistake, you're an idiot. Learn! This applies to who you date, a job, your friends, and items you purchase, anything.

Your gut is the greatest barometer of right or wrong. If not now, it will be one day.

Look, I have done multiple projects, jobs, relationships, interests, schooling in my life in which I did not succeed in society's sense of the word. I have done things, truly worked hard, and was not successful—an amazing life lesson. This is important for everyone to hear because that happens too in life. It is not all unicorns, rainbows, and lavender water out there. The perspective I have now almost makes my failures seem all right.

Failure is a funny thing, though, because most people tend to think of it as a negative in life, especially when we are young. I know the mental blocks it causes in our youth, and it can be paralyzing. I have been there, too, in a variety of situations. And each time the feeling afterward is pretty similar; you feel like a can of smashed lug nuts. If there is no one there to support you, even worse.

But failure is awesome, like, earth-shattering good because all these failures make us who we will become down the road. They lay the foundation, failure brick by failure brick, for the successes we will have later in life.

Sounds crazy but think of your life like building a house. Without the foundation (failures), you would have nothing sturdy on which to build your home (your life). And, at the very least, your failure means you are trying; you are not being stagnant.

I fail every day. I, literally, fail every day. It's not because I suck; it's because I keep trying.

Keep failing!

THE REMINDERS

Take risks. They don't always pay off, but take risks, especially when you are young.

Without failure, how can you appreciate success?

Your gut is the greatest barometer you will ever have.

8 Love Simply

My job on this day was to simply deliver cremated remains to a local cemetery so that they could be interred per the family's wishes. At times, families wish to bring the remains themselves, but today I was asked to deliver them on behalf of a family.

I pulled into the cemetery on this early morning with the hint of dew in the air and its moisture still coating the green grass. As I drove in, I noticed something odd in the distance. One of those low beach chairs, the ones only slightly raised above the sand that, depending on your weight, have your backside almost touching the ground. In this low-set chair sat a man in a jacket, maybe a windbreaker, wearing a hat. He looked to be sleeping, or maybe relaxing as the sun slowly rose on this September morning.

I drove by and saw the man was not sleeping at all, just deep in thought staring at a gravestone.

As I exited my car and headed into the office, I looked back at the man. He was unmoved from his trance-like stare. I couldn't keep my eyes off him, wondering if he was okay.

"What's with the guy in the lawn chair?" I asked Mary, who

was at the front desk as I signed the necessary paperwork documenting this transfer of precious cargo. I couldn't help but ask. Mary looked up at me and stopped.

Then, a smile slowly crossed her face. "That is Mr. Tenant."

Okay.

"He's here every day."

"Every day?" I said surprised.

"Every day. He lost his wife a few years ago, and he comes here every day to be with her."

"Like—"

"EVERY day! Some days he waters. Some days he trims. Some days he washes. Some days he just sits. He said she was the only true love of his life. He said he would be with her until the end."

Tears filled her eyes. I barely knew this woman, and we were standing before each other thinking the exact same thing. How profoundly beautiful.

"Thank you." I smiled at her.

"You are welcome." Mary smiled back knowing this was so much more than a delivery of one family's precious cargo for me.

I left the building and stopped. Mr. Tenant was still sitting there with his wife.

What I thought was a simple delivery turned into a day with so much greater meaning than I could have ever learned elsewhere: the enduring power of love.

WE ALL LOVE DIFFERENTLY

If you were lucky enough to fall in love, congratulations. It is not easy. Love is a many splendored thing—and a very complicated thing.

I would like to first point out that we all love quite differently. I can see this in my own family, the family in which I grew up, my in-laws, and various friends and their families. There is no correct way to love. We should simply understand we all love differently.

I have broken loving down into a few parts: how we innately love within us and at what stage we are in our lives when we love. In the end, I can guarantee you this: Your love road, like your life road, will get rocky at multiple points along the way; no one is immune. But having the love of a partner will help ease the bumps in your road.

By "how" we love, I simply mean how we, as humans, innately love others. For example, I happen to be an over-the-top hugger with my sons. I am a mad snuggler. I like my sons close, and I love to hold their hands.

My wife likes her space. She loves our boys no less; we simply love differently.

While not all encompassing, I see four generic types of ways we innately love as humans:

There are the huggers of the world. The people who feel from the heart, who are super expressive, and you can feel it in their full body embrace. When you get a real hug from someone you love, you know it. It is not for everyone, but when you are embraced by someone, it sends a warm feeling through your body.

The "little bits." I will love you like a hugger, but not all the time. I still need my space and I don't need to be all in, 100 percent of the time. A solid person who knows their boundaries and the extent to which they can regularly commit. It is a more even-keeled person who, most likely, is highly organized and efficient.

The "don't touch me, but I love you" person who will prepare you a lovely meal, take care of you, send you a card on every occasion, but who doesn't exude the warm fuzzy from every pore. "Just know she loves you, honey."

And, of course, the "I love no one except [INSERT inanimate object, pet, job, hobby]." Those emotionally detached from other humans of the world because, well, because it is easier that way. Again, not to be frowned upon outright, they simply see their priorities in the world as separate and distinct from human love.

It is understanding this basic premise, and the reality of it, from where we should all form the basis of our understanding of love.

Scientific, right?

Once we understand we all love differently, we must also understand there are various stages of love in our lives: Your first love or puppy love. The first time you fall in love when you are in middle school or high school and that person breaks your heart, goes out with your best friend, and tells everyone you smelled like Fritos. The abject pain one feels from that love is like no other feeling in the world.

Heartbroken!

Another stage of love is the high school daze and the amazing friends you ran with. For me, going for "walks" at the middle school, having beers at the Yascos' house, making out on the golf course, the endless parties in the McAllisters' basement, the Murphys' sun porch, foolin' around in neighbors' backyards, midnight movies at The Rome, skinny-dippin' in public pools. These were the times when we were so hopped up on estrogen, testosterone, REO Speedwagon, and Miller High Life that it felt like there wasn't a care in the world or a finish line because all that fun would never end.

As our lives rolled on there were the periodic remembrances of days gone by that were triggered by some modern-day reminder, and we wanted to simply be dropped back in that moment in time singing "Baba O'Riley" at the top of our lungs, locked arm-in-arm with the forty other drunk kids from the football party at the Devine house in the fall of 1982.

But I digress.

You then "matured" to college love, which only got a little raunchier (via more alcohol and anesthetics) and was much more temporal ("Heck, the semester is almost over; I won't have to see them again until the school begins again in the fall.").

And finally, the post-collegiate love, which is a little more mature in that you wear nicer clothes and can be found less easily on campus, but much of the same carnage was only exacerbated by greater disposable income and, hopefully, a steady job.

But there comes a time in life when you need to grow up.

This is the difficult part for many men and women because there is so much excitement in the first few meetings with a person, the sneaking around, the passion, the heat—in sum, the dance.

If we are truly being honest, there is nothing like the anticipation of seeing if your feelings will be returned and the chemical reaction of that first kiss—endorphin magic! It cannot be minimized, it is addictive, and for those of you who have dated a lot, I get the runner's high of it all.

But once you are married, hopefully, the "love" becomes the

bigger thing. There is still the passion, but it is a different, calmer, more reserved, less knee-jerk-type of passion.

And how can life ever be like it was when you were younger? It can't. Period. Exclamation point!

To love simply is the mature love of marriage and being older. I hope you have had those previous times in high school, college, and the real world; otherwise, you might not be ready to love simply.

But loving simply does not mean settling. Loving simply means you care a little less about the superficial things of young love: the size of things, the shape of things, the height and weight of things.

The reality is, boobs sag, grandma panties are more comfortable than thongs, and flannel pjs are simply, well, warmer.

Now, don't get me wrong. To keep it fresh, I'll dress up like Spartacus and my wife will don the naughty seventh arrondissement nursemaid's costume here and again, but we aren't as diabolical about sex as we once were: "Honey, I'd love to give you a handy, but I hurt my wrist in spin class today so could you help yourself?"

Loving simply means you understand your partner had a tough day with the kids, or at work, and you give them a pass, even if you are in the mood. You understand that together you brought three beautiful children into the world and that sometimes your needs need to go to the back of the bus.

Now, it can't always be like that because, occasionally, you need to be first. But loving simply means subjugating your needs for the greater good of the entire family considering the history you have with this person.

I know some marriage professionals may think I am an idiot or a ticking time bomb or whatever, but it's my book, so kiss my ass.

And sometimes shit gets super real at our house.

As we all know, most of us American families with young children are completely overscheduled; the parents are running from one practice to another; and then we lay our heads down and Dad wants some and Mom wants to go to sleep. Sometimes there's a fight with words like, "I am not your blow-up doll" (actually heard that one), or "I want to be romanced" (that one too).

Sometimes you just both fall asleep because it's easier than the confrontation. I know it's not healthy, just being honest.

It is sometimes difficult for a dad to buy into the "nonsexual touching," as my wife calls it. "Everything I do does not have to lead to sex," or so I am told. Women like that. The problem is, I am just too damn stressed, and having sex would help me sleep better so can't you just play along, and I'll get you back to *Real Housewives of Beverly Hills* before that Tide commercial ends.

I am gifted that way.

This is a perfect microcosm of how "married" life and "dating" life are, oh, so very different.

"OUR" MISCARRIAGES

I started to know about loving simply very early in my marriage when my wife and I experienced a couple of miscarriages in between the births of our sons. The doctor told us Angie had a "misshapen uterus." Now, not knowing much about uteruses myself, it didn't take Stephen Hawking to figure out that didn't sound particularly excellent.

I saw the look in my wife's eyes as the doctor explained to us why it might be difficult to have more children. My wife looked over at me with tears filling her eyes. I knew exactly what she was thinking. She knew I always wanted to be a dad with a whole brood. I would always say, "I want six kids," at every family function after our engagement. I could see in her eyes this vulnerability, this longing to be able to give me all that I wanted in life, what we had talked about on numerous occasions, and now a doctor was going to tell us that might not happen.

I simply reached over and held her hand.

I looked back at the doctor and recited my best *Dumb and Dumber* line: "So, you're telling me there's a chance?"

The doctor forced a smile and nodded, but really looked at me like, "You're an idiot."

Apparently, she liked the movie too.

When we went home, there was much crying and embracing. There were talks of Angie's fears.

I listened.

I listened and reassured her this wouldn't stop us and, trying to be light, said something stupid and male-centric like, "Just think of all the practice we get to keep doing."

But, in reality, I was scared too. We had Hudson. He was healthy. He was a light unto our lives. And if we could not have any more children, we would have been blessed with our beautiful firstborn boy.

But I was scared. I was really scared. I was scared for me. I was scared for my wife.

I thought about my best friend, John. After his first born, he and his wife decided to adopt. It was a long, arduous, and expensive process. They live in Maine and made the trek halfway around the world to Hunan Province to adopt a baby girl, who was left on an orphanage doorstep. These people, this couple from Maine, went across the globe to give a child a chance. In my selfish moment of thinking about myself and my fears, I thought about my friend's selfless act of love and how difficult that must have been for them.

Or was it the exact opposite? Total excitement about this brave new world they were getting involved in.

As it turned out for them, it was definitely the latter, and Jenna Mooch is taking names and crushin' it every step of the way.

So, taking my "woe is me" moment and looking at another situation, I refocused on us. That, for me, was the moment when I knew the depth of our love. Our first of many tests. If the Lord, or body chemistry, or fate, or whatever, decided we would not have any more children, then so be it, I tried to convince myself.

But really, I wanted Hud to have brothers or sisters to play with and more little feet running around our home. I wanted the insanity it all brings, the different personalities, the whining, the sleepless nights, the worrying, the endless diapers, the sleep deprivation, the sickness, the vomiting, the exhaustion, the poop, the endless poop and its manifold shapes, consistencies, and discovery places—I wanted it all.

Be careful what you wish for.

But my desires, while real, weren't important.

The unfair paradox is that this is generally perceived as a female issue simply because "she" has the anatomy to carry a child. What if it was me? What if someone told me my body couldn't produce children?

What would you do? How would you react? Is your love that strong?

My wife was hurting, and I could see it. But this was not a "she" issue, this was a "we" issue.

I gently sat her down as I could see her mind going through the various incarnations of "what ifs" that only the human mind could iterate: "What if I'm sterile?" "What if Hud had no one to play with?" "What if we really couldn't have any more kids?" "What if, what if, what—"

I stopped her.

"I am in love with you. We will get through this together. You and me, and me and you. We have each other."

I think she liked to hear that.

Honestly, I surprised myself hearing the words come out of my mouth that evening because I knew I wasn't that strong. I knew what I wanted; I knew what my own mind was capable of saying and what it was capable of doing. But my love for my wife overrode that.

REALITY BITES

And look, the last reality about loving simply is that you are not as pretty/handsome as you were when you were younger.

True story.

You may think you are killin' it in that new outfit, but the reality is any guy or girl would have liked you more ten years younger. Your body was tighter, gravity worked with, not against, you, your hair was more plentiful, muscles tauter, your skin tighter.

That is simply the reality.

I know, I get it, you eat right, you go to the gym daily, the young boys/girls look at you, you buy the best moisturizers, the trendiest clothes, you're crushin' it.

But you're older. Nice looking and in shape, but older.

And lest, for a moment, you think I am harping on the women. Men, more so. But for some reason we think we age more gracefully; operative word here is *think*. You might think that dye camouflaging those grays makes you look younger, and you can still wear that muscle shirt because your arms are still, what, lean?

Yeah, not so much. A forty-year-old dude in a muscle shirt is still a forty-year-old dude in a muscle shirt. Our bodies age.

And now for a super-real sidebar:

Vegas. Twenty-year-old drunk and thrashing in a pool. Very cool.

Forty-year-olds doing the same. Not so cool.

Fifty-year-old. Put your damn Tommy Bahama back on.

End of sidebar.

When we get married, we tend to think in a cloud of wedded bliss. But love, marriage, life really, is never a slow trajectory upward with Moet and rose petals each step of the way up:

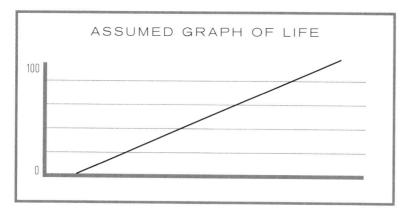

Start at zero when you get married and SHAZAM! a smooth rocket ship ride straight into the blissful stratosphere.

Record scratch! Love/marriage/life is filled with incessant peaks and valleys, and your resiliency to weather those peaks and valleys is what makes you who you are.

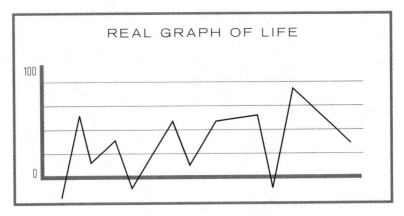

The difficult part to comprehend is that there are not always accolades for weathering the storms of life. There is not always family around to say great job, a mom or dad, grandparent or friend to give you kudos for surviving the valleys. This is where a spouse or partner can really help. You weather life together. We are stronger together.

This is the good stuff.

Look, I just believe in the institution of togetherness; the institution of marriage sounds so corporate, mundane, and religious. And maybe the grass isn't always greener on the other side. Different person, same problems.

Sometimes it takes a lot of inward reflection to realize that I am not Bezos, Adonis, Einstein, Mister Rogers, and the Dalai Lama rolled into one.

My wife seems to see that much more clearly than do I.

Love. Just do it…simply.

IN SUM

There is nothing like the intoxication of the first few meetings with another human being to whom you are attracted. If only they could bottle that. But that's simply not the reality of life. At some point, that white-hot heat has to end. And while dating is unequivocally fun, the truly good stuff, like aged whiskey, wine, or cheese (sorry, I was thirsty and hungry when I wrote this) happens over time.

We can never recapture the times of our youth no matter how hard we try. That's why they are called memories. It's not settling, it's maturing. And doing it together is pretty good too.

THE REMINDERS

Women are superior.

Love evolves over time.

Listening is the greatest gift we have.

Love/marriage/life is never a rocket ride straight up; it always has peaks and valleys.

9 Become a Familionaire

DEFINITION: *fa-MILL-yun-air* (noun) a person
who is rich in moments with their family.

THE MATRIARCH

A large family with tons of kids in our town was active in all reaches of the community. Had been for many years. Actually, for over a century. Schools and streets were named after them. You know the type.

I had befriended one of the daughters in our local Chamber of Commerce. We struck up a nice friendship with our sarcastic banter. That's how it usually happens with friends. You see something in them you like.

I was extremely honored when she wanted me to take care of her mother—not if, but when, she passed. She was under hospice care, and the family anticipated her death shortly.

The call came in the dead of night. I quietly got up, showered, and put on my suit while stepping over a gaggle of sons around my bedroom. I called my friend and told her I was on the way. She warned me there were a lot of people at the home. I said I would be right over.

This was the Roman Catholic matriarch of a large middle-class family. Now to say it like that makes it sound somewhat regal and snooty, but what I simply mean is this woman was grandmother to a bunch of grandchildren (in excess of twenty) and mother to a lot of children (nine, I believe).

I arrived to find the living room strewn with kids, girlfriends, aunts, uncles, all holding hands, hugging, talking as the outsider in the suit arrived in the darkness.

"Hi, I'm Chris from the funeral home." Yup, as cheery as a summer day. Doesn't everyone want to run over and hug the guy who's gonna wheel grandma out of her home feet first? You get the idea.

A couple of alphas rolled over and introduced themselves as the sons and looked me over as if I had committed a heinous crime with a rusty butter knife to one of their kinfolk in front of them.

I am used to the scrutiny by this point, so I extended my hand and looked them directly into their eyes, confident, professional, strong in my uncertainty.

"Yah, my sister said you might come by," said the smaller, clearly more volatile of the two. People in the midst of extreme incidents of stress tend to be ruder and more hair-trigger personalities. By now, I get it and am not offended. You add in lack of sleep, improper eating, a drink or two, and you can easily understand why people act the way they do.

The tough part of the job is sussing out the personalities and power structures within the families at a moment's notice.

Luckily, my friend called to me from the back of the room, rushed over, and gave me a big, warm hug. This instantly allayed the fears of others in the room about the "grandma taker."

After our greetings and a few formalities, I asked if I could see her mom to assess how we were going to remove her from the home. Many people understandably do not think of this when caring for someone. I have removed people from many precarious positions like toilets, showers, corners of beds, backyards, you name it, always after the fire department, police, or coroner have given their okay.

As an aside, let me explain how this works. The funeral home is never the first call when someone is suspected to have died at home. This is distinguished from someone dying at the hospital or in a care home. As I mentioned earlier, if under hospice care at home, the hospice nurse will pronounce the death, then call the funeral home.

If someone dies at home in other circumstances, 911 should be called first. Once the officer does their preliminary investigation, they will call the coroner if they don't understand why this person has died. If the coroner does not take the body with them back to the county morgue, they will instruct the family to call a funeral home. This means they already know why the person died.

If the coroner decides to take the body, this means they have a question about the circumstances under which this person died or didn't understand why the person died. They will need to do an autopsy on the body to determine a cause of death. After that is done, and this takes a number of days up to weeks, depending on the jurisdiction in which you live, the coroner will notify the family and tell them to call a funeral home to pick up the body. This is a rudimentary roadmap of what to do when someone dies at home.

In this situation, hospice had pronounced. With a houseful of family and grandma still in her bed where she died, I went to the back bedroom to find another roomful of people surrounding the matriarch. There were literally daughters and grandchildren on either side of the bed still crying and holding their grandmother's hand.

I said, "I can come back."

My friend looked at me and said, "No, it's time. We waited to call you. All came who wanted to come, and we have all said our last goodbyes."

I walked out with my friend as her brothers walked up. I explained exactly what was going to happen and how a coworker and I would remove their mother. I explained how many families chose to avoid this part as we place their mother in a plastic bag (to prevent leakage that often happens with bodies at end of life), slide her onto the removal cot, and cover her to remove her from her home.

They asked me not to cover their mother's face. The family did not want to see her like that as we took her from her home.

I was in a strange place here. I understood they did not want a sheet pulled over their mother's face, but at the same time, it would be alarming if neighbors or cars passing by witnessed an uncovered body leaving a home. Most times, we acquiesce to the family's request.

I nodded my understanding and went outside to meet my coworker, and we made our plan of attack. I explained there were a lot of people in the home. He nodded his understanding.

"No, like a real lot."

By the time we had walked back in, the scene was unreal. Normally, a grieving spouse is there when I arrive to remove a life partner, a few of their children, some family, but never so many family members from two, maybe three generations.

It was majestic really. Everyone was now standing arm-in-arm next to one another lining the rooms and hallways to grandma's bedroom. It was a human pathway to the back room that they had organized out of love, respect, and honor.

I could clearly see the effect this woman had on her family. This is what it meant to be a famillionaire.

Obviously, she was loved. But this was more than that—if there is such a thing. This is what family is all about, however you define family. There were blood relatives, there were friends, there were long-time neighbors. This was goodness, this was respect, this was a ton of love of generations of one family in one place and at one time. For me this is what it is all about. The great reminder. Looking around the room that night brought it all into clearer focus for me.

This is what I want. This is how I want it all to end. This is what drives my each and every movement from this day forward. I don't need this car, or those clothes, or this house, or that job.

This...this is it!

All these people focused on our every movement to take their beloved grandma, mother, and friend out of her home for the last time.

When we got to her room with the cot, many chose to stay and witness our care for their mother. We try to be as careful as humanly possible, but honestly there isn't an easy way of getting someone onto a portable gurney in a graceful manner. To their credit, a few family members wanted to help, and truly did.

We took her from her home for the last time. The smaller brother who had studied me so closely came over and told me he would follow me back to the funeral home. He wanted to honor his mother by following her to her final resting place. In reality, I knew he wanted to see where she was going.

Unusual, yes, but of course we allow this.

When I got back to the funeral home, he asked if he could come in and follow her into the cooler. This hadn't happened before. Again, of course, I allowed it. To do otherwise would be tantamount to my hiding something from the family.

I knew he wanted to judge the cleanliness of the place and see exactly where Mom was going. I did what I had done hundreds of times before and placed his mother on a shelf in the cooler. He, all the while, watching my every step and looking around everywhere judging, smelling, watching my every movement.

I closed the cooler door and he stood there staring at me. It got awkward.

Then, he extended his hand. "Thank you. Thank you for taking care of my mother."

"You are very welcome. I am honored your family entrusted me."

He kept staring at me and nodded. Then he turned and left.

Family is complicated.

But family is everything in this world, however you define it.

MODERN FAMILY?

I believe all of us with children may have it wrong.

Does this sound familiar? Wake up. School. Practice. Homework. Bed. Repeat.

We are living *Groundhog Day*, the movie.

On the weekends, Mom and Dad split up and each takes a child to various games, practices, or travel tournaments, maybe sleeping over in some rando town holding a tournament, or maybe getting home in time to sleep in your own bed and do it all again the next day.

We do this for three seasons a year—and summer is even busier.

I spoke to a friend in the hotel business. His company builds and operates moderately priced hotels around the country: Residence Inns, Comfort Suites, Days Inns. I asked him the naive question: "I get that you have business travelers all week, but do you hear crickets on the weekends?"

He smiled wryly and said, "Nope, travel ball. We get families from everywhere, in every sport, staying for our two-night minimums with a waffle breakfast, year-round."

I love waffles, but what are we all doing?

Why does an eight-year-old need to be on a traveling basketball team that keeps you away from your spouse and your child away from their siblings for most of the weekend? Not to mention practices during the week. And I am not preaching here. I am guilty of coaching all three of my sons' basketball teams in one year, placing me on the cusp of a nervous breakdown and a heart attack with a side of aneurysm in the process.

Now here's a refreshing piece of reality. There are, and generally always have been, a finite number of slots in professional sports and, most likely, your child will not be one of them.

Harsh, but true.

I believe we are so caught up in the competition of our suburban lives that we are losing track of the greatness and simplicity of life. The times spent imagining, creating, or playing alone or with one's own siblings, board games or simply playing with army men, dolls, or figurines.

What happened to that?

The greatest memories of my childhood were playing with my brother in what we called The Diggins—literally a dirt mound, with uprooted tree roots, under an old oak tree in our backyard. My brother and I could play in the dirt for days with our army men and trucks. We would pretend to have battles, create scenarios, and talk to each other in a variety of commanding and supporting military voices.

We would be out there all day, maybe come in for lunch or a snack, but we always left our army men set up so we could return and seamlessly pick up where we left off. The shade of the tree would provide a calm coolness to those humid summer days. We would come in with dirt under our nails and filth on our clothes, but those were the days of summer, the days you were supposed to come home dirty. I look back and think about the unmitigated joy we shared together just, well, just playing in dirt.

Now, I look at my kids and wonder.

They are kids of the tech era and their play is very different from mine. My wife and I have often sent them outside to just "go and play," and, sadly, they don't know what to do. I remember us watching them from inside our home, seeing them struggling to play with cars in the dirt; my wife and I watching like two scientists in a lab studying how rats react to different stressors. It was really quite tragic.

And what do we expect really, with Dolby quality surround sound, technicolor effects, and lifelike avatars running around blasting enemies on 42-inch HD screens whether it's Fortnite, Rainbow Siege, or Call of Duty.

Showing them the first video game of Pong I played was futile. "What's the point of this, Dad?"

I often look at them when they are sitting around me, all wearing their Beats headphones, and slowly drift off to those endless summer days with my brother. There were times when we were playing in the dirt I would just stop and furtively focus on him as he talked out loud the battles our army men were in. He was older, so I was seeing how he would use his imagination and accompanying word choices. I would listen to his voice and the intonations he would use and try to follow the stories he was creating with his mind and words.

Invariably, he would catch me watching him and just stop and stare at me. My eyes would quickly dart away, and I would riff off of his last words, like some neophyte jazz musician in a smoke-filled nightclub on Bleecker Street, seamlessly adding to his stories or spinning more elaborate yarns with different scenarios that would extend our imaginary play.

As I look back at those days, those were the times of our lives. The times I felt closest to my brother. We were different, for sure, but playing together we could be best friends for hours, days on end. To this very day, I truly believe that is at the root of our existing bond for one another.

With my own sons, I realize I can't force them to have fun the way I did, but isn't it really an indictment of me? I bought them the Xbox and the iPad. Am I the problem?

Of course, I am, I am their parent. The responsibility lies with me. But after a hard day's work and my wife playing bus driver for the children, we are tired too.

You feel me, right? Is this what life is? I am no better than you, and, in many ways, I am way worse. But we need to stop.

Our job as parents is to give our children a solid foundation so that they, in turn, will grow to lead a happy and healthy life, right? I am not trying to raise the next LeBron. I want to teach my children how to love. To be kind. To cope. And how to get along with others.

But most of all I want to teach them about family. About where they came from and what matters most in life. So, for me, it comes down to a simple question, and this is where the funeral guy sticks his head in again and asks, Who do you want at your deathbed?

I believe this is the threshold question in becoming a famillionaire. Do you want your family there? Maybe a few close friends?

These are the people that matter most in life. Sure, your brother rubs you the wrong way and he can get under your skin like no other, but he is still your brother. And you came from the same blood, right? You are family and family is not always pretty.

Or maybe you don't want anyone around; maybe you don't want to put your loved ones through that. I get that too because the end is never pretty.

Please take these words from me today as if I am your own personal funeral Yoda. The end is never pretty, and, oftentimes, it is brutal.

For those of you who swabbed the inside of your loved one's mouth with those lollipop-like sticks with sponges on the end of them so they didn't dehydrate because they could no longer swallow liquids; for those of you who have placed Chapstick on the lips of your loved ones because they couldn't lift their arms to do so themselves; for those of you who have moisturized and rotated your loved one's body to prevent bed sores; and for those of you who have propped another pillow behind your loved one's back or neck to prevent their lungs from filling with bodily liquids so they didn't drown in an unpleasant death right before your eyes...

For all of you...God bless you. And for those of you who want no part of it, I get that too.

But I want to be there. I will be there.

Why? Because our loved ones need us, and they want us there.

My Opa was the proudest man I have ever known, always dressed to a T, clean-shaven, and smelling of Old Spice. Near the end of his life, in the depths of his illness one Christmas Eve, I slept in the same room with him because he couldn't be alone anymore. In the middle of the night, he pinballed his way to the bathroom, bouncing off doorframes like padded bumpers, an ancient pinball wizard playing a cruel end-of-life game.

And when he went to the bathroom, I had to wipe him because he would forget.

I don't tell you this because I want you to think I am special, some amazing kid with a special talent. I tell you this because I was simply a grandson in love with his grandfather, an average kid in every way. I have no idea what made me act like that in his time of need. I had no training, no special gift or calling.

It was just love.

So think about this. Who do you want there? Is it better that it is someone, a nurse, a hospice worker, someone who does not know you the way your family does? Or is it better if it is your grandson? And could your grandson do it? Would you want your grandson to do it? Would you want him to remember you like that?

I will tell you this. I will tell you this with every fiber of truth in my soul, being around my grandfather as he was dying gave me a far greater appreciation for life than anything I had ever done up to that point in my existence.

ANYTHING!

I felt closer to him in his sunset than when his mind was sharp as a tack, and we had the greatest grandfather-grandson love affair when he was of sound mind.

And why?

Because he needed me. I knew he needed me when I looked into his cloudy eyes. I knew it. Don't get me wrong, my Opa had amazing women who took care of him (Mary and Bridgette are gods in my family's eyes), but that I could play a small part in his care gave me empathy, the ability to understand the feelings of another, not sympathy, when you share the feelings of another.

Sympathy is easy. I'm talking empathy, when you put yourself in their shoes. He was me. I imagined me being there in that moment, and I knew how much I loved him, and how much he loved me and that, as proud a human being as he was, he would have wanted no one else more than me there for him. I knew as clear as the sun will rise tomorrow, he wanted me there.

So, think…

Who do you really want there?

DIVORCE AND BEING A FAMILLIONAIRE

But doesn't divorce mess up this whole famillionaire thing?

No. No different at all, maybe even more important.

Depending on which statistic you believe, about half the marriages in America (and the world) end up in divorce. I am hoping that number is high, but I believe it based on what I see around us. This is no holier-than-thou speech nor is it an indictment of divorce. I simply empathize with those who have gone through it or are going through it. And I especially empathize with the children of those parents. Some of our dearest friends have gone through divorce, and it stinks all around.

I can't even imagine dating at this age, when I grew up in a world of meeting in bars, and we have now transformed to a society of Match.com, Bumble, Tinder, and the like. I am definitely not as handsome, nor as thin, as I once was, and I am fairly certain my snoring would be endearing to no one at all out there.

Marriages break up for a variety of reasons. I often say you have no idea what goes on, or doesn't go on, behind closed doors. I think infidelity, drinking, and drug use are hard to overcome in a marriage, but there are certainly those warriors who have battled through it.

Respect.

My parents have been married sixty years, and Angie's folks fifty-six. We have a lot to live up to. While I do not profess to know the trials and tribulations of my in-laws, I can unequivocally say my parents' marriage could not have been easy. I love my parents equally, but they are both stubborn Germans at heart, and unless you know a German, you have no idea what I mean. That's probably a horrible indictment of my forefathers, and I should narrow "Germans" to only my mom's and dad's families, but you get my point.

I have seen them fight and be mad at each other, but they have stuck at it through everything and I am grateful.

I don't know the divorced life, and I don't want to know it. I am sorry for families that do. The key is this: Becoming a famillionaire is surrounding yourself with those people you consider family. In no way does it have to mean your own blood; there are no rules.

Family is how you define it, and we all define family in our own unique way. Who will line the hallways when the funeral guy comes to remove you after you have died at home? Who do you want there?

IN SUM

I am simply advocating for a throwback to a simpler way of life, for getting off the Habitrail society tells us to jump on and stay on. Don't buy in. The good stuff is right here in front of our own faces, right within our own homes, it's as clear as day. We all need less in our lives, way less. We can do this.

THE REMINDERS

Slow down. You move too fast. You gotta make the morning last.

———

Revel in the simplicity of family togetherness.

———

Who do you want at your deathbed?

———

It takes no money; your children just want you.

———

Family is how you define it.

———

10 Make a Few Good Friends

"Hey, Chris, we got a little problem."

The phrase every funeral home owner loves to hear.

"You gotta come see this," said Ken, the funeral arranger.

I followed Ken to the chapel where we were holding a memorial service that evening. The casket was open displaying a young man in his thirties, who had died under suspicious circumstances.

I walked up to the casket and saw the man lying there, as he should be, nothing seemingly amiss.

"Looks good to me."

"Open the bottom of the casket," Ken said.

As most of you know, the top half the casket is usually open, or up, to display the top half of the body. The bottom half of the casket is generally closed to cover the body waist down with a casket spray usually sitting atop the wood veneer of the casket.

I opened the casket to see what Ken was alluding to and saw—

A joint, a few condoms, a bottle of Jack, and...a Glock 9mm.

"What the—"

Ken said, "I didn't—"

"Who the—"

"Me!" I heard a deep voice shout from the back of the chapel.

Ken and I turned to see a brick, multifamily house of a man standing 6 feet 5 inches tall, at least 260 pounds, with tats covering more of his exposed body than skin on my own.

"Back off!" the enormous man exclaimed.

Ken scurried off like a scared ferret. "I'll let you two be alone."

Thanks, Ken.

The dude marched up to me with an extra bounce in his step. "Who are you?" he shouted aggressively.

"I'm the owner."

"Of what?"

"The a…the funeral home."

"Oh, nice to meet you, man." He extended his hand in an immediately friendlier tone.

I shook it. "Charmed."

"Charmed. That's funny. You English?"

"German."

"Gracias," he replied nonplussed.

"I think we're getting a little off track here."

"What's the problem, brah?"

"There seems to be gun in the casket."

"And a joint, a bottle of Jack, and a few condoms," he clarified astutely.

"I can't have a gun in the funeral home."

"It's in the casket."

"Which is in the funeral home," I quickly replied.

"Brah."

He stared at me for a beat like come on, dude.

"I can't—"

"It's not loaded."

A welcomed consolation.

"I wasn't gonna do that until everyone left," he clarified.

"Sir—"

"Chill! My homie needs a few things to keep him comfortable where he's going."

"I'm fairly certain he won't be needing any of those things in heaven, brotha."

"Who said anything about heaven?" he replied with a smirk.

Touché. Only a friend would know.

A BEST FRIEND

I met the best friend I have in life at law school.

John was an older guy from Maine who had a real job working for the Norfolk Naval Shipyard in Virginia Beach, after graduating from Maine Maritime Academy. He worked as a field engineer doing shipboard troubleshooting on nuclear surface ships with the highest security clearance. We met on a basketball court at law school, and after we played, he affectionately asked another guy, "Who's the asshole from New York?"

Thirty years later, we are still best friends.

Everyone in his hometown knew him and seemingly always has. He was a big dude, around 6 feet 4 and 280 pounds, a larger-than-life figure. Each year, we would spend New Year's vacations together, and we would often joke how he waves and honks his car horn to everyone as we would drive down Main Street, like the mayor at a Fourth of July parade. I loved going there and being in his world where there was an amazing sense of community, great people, and characters—a real slice of Americana.

John's dad is the nicest man in the world: kind, gentle, and an avid student of the stock market. His mom, known to a select few as Gurgs, was one of the most interesting women to talk to. She was well versed in southern Maine history and horticulture and a solid judge of character. Gurgs made us massive breakfasts on New Year's morning featuring her world-famous popovers. She died a few years ago after some unhealthy years. I know the void John feels. A great American woman.

John was born with partially clubbed feet; everything below his ankle was not fully developed. But despite walking on the outsides of his feet, he played sports, walked pretty regular for a big dude; in many ways, he was an anomaly for a person with his condition. After graduation from law school, his feet started to turn in so badly he would wake up and see the bottoms of his feet. In 1999 the condition got so bad, he was confined to a wheelchair and forced to buy a special van.

But he never missed a beat.

In 2000, the doctors tried a fairly radical surgery, breaking every bone in his foot and tried to reconstruct it.

It didn't work.

In 2003, it got so bad they amputated his leg. A life-altering event.

I remember him describing the sensation of his leg still being attached, his mind tricking him. He had to learn to walk again.

It was frustrating. He had to push. He had nurses, doctors, and therapists, family and friends, and an amazing wife and kids, all who helped him, all heroic people. But, at the end of the day, it was just him with no leg. We would talk about the loss, and we cried together. I know I cried alone. I was scared. This was my best friend in the whole world.

I thought, how is he going to deal with this? How does one rebound from such a life-altering event?

His wife? His children? How would anyone?

I'll tell you how. He dug deep. He dug real frickin' deep. He worked. He pounded. He was a warrior. A modern-day warrior in the true sense of the word.

He always showed a smile, even with gnarled teeth.

Then...

He got an infection in his back that temporarily paralyzed him. Then, a second infection that almost killed him. And finally, in 2004, they amputated his other leg.

Double amputee and he wasn't even forty-three.

As God as my witness, I have never heard him complain or use his handicap as a crutch once. Not once.

You think you got it bad? Shut your mouth, pick yourself up, and keep frickin' pounding!

We are grown men and despite 3,066 miles separating us, we speak on the phone five times a week, much to our wives' chagrin. I cannot express how much I enjoy simply hearing his voice every day. It brings me comfort. Sometimes it's quick, sometimes it's for an hour.

I look forward to our talks.

As a grown man, it is a blessing to have a trusted confidante with whom I can share everything, and nothing. I realize how lucky I am to have a friend whom I can talk to and not feel weird about it being almost every day. It is weird to some. I don't care.

That is a friend. John is my friend. John knows how much I love him. I tell John I love him a lot. John is a warrior.

I named my middle son after him.

A "TRUE" FRIEND

So it got me to thinking about friends. What is a friend? What is a true friend?

There are so many people we call friends. People we see at our kids' school, church, go to parties with and have fun, people we can call and go out to dinner with on any given weekend. Those are friends, and most people have many of them. People with whom you have a great time with when you are out. Ya know, friends.

But isn't a real friend, a true friend, someone you want in your space, your home? Someone with whom you can really talk, and not merely about the superficial stuff: sports, kids, weather? These are the people you let see you with no makeup on, in your shorts or ratty T-shirts, the people for whom there are no pretenses. The people you just enjoy being with in a relaxed atmosphere.

When I am with John, I am just me. I don't believe he cares about how much money I have, what car I drive, or the family stock from whence I came. I think he likes me for me, warts and all, as the saying goes. I know he would help me if I were down, as I would help him in any situation. It is comforting knowing

I can pick up the phone and talk to him; sometimes it is just comforting to pick up the phone and hear his voice. We have established a brotherhood. We have established a true friendship and a love for one another.

Some of my fondest memories are when neither of us had a cent to our name and we would get together over New Year's. We would watch football and talk away the weekend. Often, we would wake up real early and go to Congdon's Donuts in Wells, get a box of donuts, and sit by the ocean. We would sit there, eat donuts, and simply look out at the ocean and watch the waves break.

It was so peaceful at early morning in January.

John would tell me of his childhood memories of playing at the beach with his family. In that instant, I could see how similar our lives were—how similar all our lives are really. Memories at the beach with our families.

I remembered how much I loved the beach with my family and how much those memories meant to me. My memories are of Cape Cod, the Townsend Dam, Pike's Falls, and Jones Beach, the places I would go with my family. I am fairly certain we didn't have much money in those times, but I never knew we had no money. We went out to eat on a special occasion, and my mom and dad cooked at our home often, but I never knew it was to save money. Nor did I even care. I was with my family, and, looking back on it, those were amazing times I will never forget.

Times I want to steal back. Moments I want to go to again and again.

The unfortunate thing about these times is, generally, we never realize how special they are until we reflect back upon them. But don't despair, that's what memories are for, that's the good stuff. That is the lifeblood of our existence.

Sitting by the ocean with John, I knew these were great times. We would lament not living closer to one another so we could "do this regularly." Those times, the times when you are together with a friend doing nothing. Just talking. Just being in each other's space, just coexisting.

Before she passed, John's mom had a painting commissioned of that exact bench where John and I would sit eating our donuts, looking out at the ocean. She gave it to me one New Year's Day.

It is my prized possession. That painting personifies true friendship to me.

IN SUM

People, these are the times of our lives. Do not bypass them for anything. There is no job, no task, no money that could ever replace these moments with friends. Take the time. Take time while people are healthy and alive, or sick, or mad, or whatever, to be with them, to laugh, to cry, to just "be" with them.

Not everyone has family who are nearby or with whom we are in touch, so true friends can easily fill that void, if a void exists. People who will put themselves on the line for you when you are down. Or at least place a Glock 9mm and some liquor in your casket.

You don't need a lot of friends, but a few true friends make life easier.

THE REMINDERS

*Honor those who have come and gone
with your happy memories.*

---

*We don't need a lot, but a few good
friends are vital for long life.*

Who can you just "be you" with?

11 Be with Self

In my role as a funeral home owner, I wanted to be different. If a surviving loved one wanted something, no matter how outlandish, I wanted to accommodate them. I figured who am I to tell them what is right or wrong at an end-of-life celebration?

One of the most unusual requests came from a mother who lost her teenage daughter to a car accident. As tragic as all deaths are, it is seemingly more so when they are young people. The mother came in with her other teenage daughter to make arrangements. After we made the arrangements, the mother said, "We have an unusual request."

"What's that?" I asked nonplussed.

"We would like to take her for a while."

"Excuse me?" I replied startled.

"We would like to drive her around town with her friends for a while. Ya know, one last joy ride."

I looked at her like, "Are you frickin' insane?"

But neither she nor her daughter was smiling back at me. They just stared back at me like puppies awaiting my approval.

"I need to check." I smiled awkwardly as I left the room.

I went to talk to the brains of the operation, our manager, Betty. She said there was no legal preclusion from a family doing what they wanted to do.

"You have got to be kidding me," I said.

Shakes of her head, "Nothing."

Astonished at this response, I walked back into the room and smiled.

"Sure." I couldn't believe my mouth said that.

And they took her. We loaded the casket in their station wagon, and they took her along with a few friends. I swear all I could think of was the movie *Weekend at Bernie's,* in which two young coworkers maneuver their dead boss so as not to spoil their vacation at a gorgeous mansion on the water.

They told me they drove around town to their old haunts: their high school parking lot, cruising the main drag, the secret places where they used to drink beers down by the river, even took her through the drive-through window at Mickey Ds.

When they finally brought her back to the funeral home, the mother was clearly coming down off an emotional high with her daughter's friends. When all the kids left, I could see the mother was now hurting.

She asked if she could stay awhile. I smiled and nodded. I had work to do in the back. We placed her daughter in a viewing room, as we usually do for families, and the mother sat with her child. She needed to be alone.

A few hours later, I stuck my head into the viewing room to make sure Mom was okay. She was just staring lovingly at her daughter, as if in a dream-like trance.

She never took her eyes of her child, but heard me come in. "I miss her."

What do I say? I'm the professional. I'm the guy to provide the right words at this moment. But I've got nothing. Parents aren't supposed to bury their children. It's just not supposed to go down like that. I have done it so many times: infants, newborns, children, and teenagers. It is horrific, the worst of the worst.

I, literally, have nothing for this woman. What? "God needed another angel?" "Only the good die young?"

Please.

"You have to close up shop, right?"

I smiled back at her. It's 7:00 p.m. and everyone is now gone. But I knew she needed more time. I could see that by the look in her eyes.

So I reached into my pocket, took the key off my keychain, and handed it to her. "Stay."

"I'm gonna stay all night," she answered gleefully.

I tried to imagine her pain, but that somehow cheapens the unfathomable loss she must have been feeling. There is no way to feel the pain in the loss of a child. None.

I went home and held my son a little tighter, tucked him in a little longer, and lay awake that night trying to imagine that woman back at my funeral home lost in her aloneness.

The job stayed with me.

And she stayed all night.

I arrived back in the morning, and she was still in the room with her daughter, now clearly exhausted, lacking sleep, naturally, looking every bit worse for the wear, hurting even worse than when I had last seen her.

I saw her pain. I felt it and realized it was about to get worse. This next moment. Now. Right here. This moment is critical. This is it. The last time a person will ever see their loved one again on this earth. I could see by the way she was looking at her daughter that she was thinking the same thing.

How do you walk away from this? Who wants to walk away from this? The moment of "I will never see you again." I've been in this situation multiple times and it is brutal for everyone involved. If it's your loved one, it goes without saying. If you work in the funeral business, there is no way you cannot relate.

She stood up and gave me a long embrace. She held me like she had known me for years, like the greatest friend she had ever known. She whispered, "Thank you. Thank you so much."

She handed me the key, kissed her daughter, and left the funeral home.

I thought of her a lot. I thought of that woman for the rest of my career. Even now, as I write this, I put myself in her shoes. I couldn't bear it. At that moment, I knew I could not make this my career. I felt too much. I feel too much.

Is that possible?

I saw her a year later in a grocery store in town. She barely recognized me when I introduced myself. She looked at me and studied my face, slowly remembering what could never be forgotten; tears slowly welled up in her eyes.

"Good man. You're a good man." And she turned and walked away.

I watched her disappear into the grocery aisle. I felt horrible. I felt really horrible. I should have just walked by her, I thought. But I brought her back. She was probably just healing, and I brought her back.

ALONE IN LA

If you knew me in high school and college, you would not describe me as a loner. In fact, I generally wanted to be with my friends, or playing sports, every single night of my existence, and preferably both in the same night. That was my life until I was thirty. I was the last person who would want to be alone, and I never was.

After law school, I chose a life of solitude, which was the complete opposite to the life I had, heretofore, led. I found what I loved to do, and it turned out to be a singular pursuit, which required being alone. Writing.

In Hollywood there was a very formulaic way to write a screenplay, a paradigm, if you will: Everyman-type protagonist starts out with a fatal flaw. An inciting incident in the first five pages builds to a first turning point at the end of that first act that catapults our unwilling hero into action, obstacles placed in front of the protagonist gradually increase in difficulty, closer and closer together to build dramatic tension, until the second turning point at the end of the second act when the audience must see there is simply no way out for our hero.

Then in the third act, at the seeming precipice of death, or surefire failure, our hero somehow miraculously pulls out an impossible sequence of events to become a better, changed, more evolved person from the one who started out on page one. That is the basic structure of most screenplays.

There, I saved you a ton of screenwriting classes.

I had written, directed, and produced a small art house film called *Black Is White* that went to a few festivals, and I was now interested in writing more Hollywood fare to pay the bills.

I know…sellout!

What I specifically loved about writing was the creative process. For me, it was to be disciplined and write for eight hours a day. The actual task of writing could take on many forms: researching, reading, outlining, and, many times, simply lying on my bed and staring at the ceiling. This was the most difficult thing to train myself to do, not because I couldn't do it, but because I constantly fought off the voice in my head telling me I was being lazy, doing nothing—the artist's quandary.

Having grown up in a German household where work ethic was everything and creativity was at a minimum (or nonexistent), this was my greatest obstacle. Once I got good at suppressing the voices in my head, I would relish the times when I laid on my bed and the creative synapses would fire like firecrackers inside my brain. I would say I was one of the best screenwriters Hollywood ever had who never sold a script. I truly believe that.

Dang, those raisins are tart!

Toward the end of my Hollywood noncareer, I was so good at outlining prior to writing a screenplay that I could write an entire script (110 pages) in three days. Now, anyone who has ever written anything knows writing is all about rewriting, but the point is I could get a script on the page fast.

I spent eleven years trying to be a writer in Hollywood. They were, at times, very lonely years. I had a few friends, guys I played basketball with, but for the most part it was a time of great solitude. I learned more about myself being alone in Los Angeles than during any other part of my life. You see, I was the child least likely to move away from Mom and Dad. In fact, when I drove my car out of my parents' driveway and headed west, I remember looking in my rearview mirror and seeing them not being all that sad. True story. I think they figured I'd be back in a month.

I drove across America in two and half days. Yes, it's possible. No, I have no good reason why. Kind of like climbing Kilimanjaro. It was just there, so I did it.

The idea of driving alone across America was scintillating. It was quiet. It was the early nineties before cell phones, but I had a car phone my father let me use to keep in touch with him. I remember him laughing as I told him each city I passed. He kept saying, "You are where? For the love of God, stop and get something to eat."

It became so much of a competition with myself that I was urinating in the Gatorade bottles as I finished them.

I nearly passed out from exhaustion somewhere outside of Boulder before laying my head down to rest.

In retrospect, I saw my journey across America as me telling myself I do not want to be alone. Let me get to Los Angeles the fastest way I know how. And yet, Los Angeles turned out to be the land of solitude for me. I grew up as a human being there. I was okay with being alone there. I didn't know anyone. I got uncomfortable. Really uncomfortable. And out of that came greatness.

Not greatness in that I sold a script for a million dollars, but rather that I became okay with being alone. See, that was my victory. I was alone as a person, and, in that solitude, I found my gift of writing (totally subjective, I understand).

IN SUM

In learning to be okay with being alone, I found confidence, maturity, and the joy of writing. I know I am more creative alone. My solitude also forced me to grow up in a way I never would have in my own comfortable bubble back home. In many ways, for me, being alone was the first step in growing up, albeit it at a very late age in life.

Now, with three sons of my own, I treasure the times I can be alone, away from the disquiet of our household, not because I don't love my family, but because I find peace in that solitude, a recharging of my brain. The peace that I am certain will keep me healthier in the long run.

THE REMINDERS

Being alone instills personal growth.

———————————

Being alone is healthy for long-term living and relationships.

———————————

Being alone enhances your creativity.

———————————

Sometimes we simply need to be alone with our thoughts.

———————————

12 Laugh

I walked into the arrangement room ready for my next family. An attractive woman, Carol, in her late sixties, and I exchanged smiles.

"I am sorry for your loss."

"Thank you. My husband and I had a lot of fun together."

"What an amazing thing to say about your spouse," I responded.

We started the normal way by taking vital statistics for the accuracy of the death certificate. It is critical that these data are exact as it will be the basis of the official document from the county or city in which the decedent has passed. The arrangement proceeded like normal as we spoke of a traditional burial, the casket, and embalming her husband for viewing.

"So, you're gonna prepare him?"

"If that is your desire, yes."

A pregnant pause. She was now looking down.

I let her have a moment clearly seeing her searching for something in her brain. Or maybe fighting back the enormity of losing her husband at such, what I consider, his young age of seventy-two.

Her chin rose slowly and her blue eyes now had the life of three smiling infants.

"I have a crazy question" (never heard that before in my funeral life and I secretly love what genuinely follows after this perfunctory phrase).

"Shoot," I said.

"Leo was a clown."

"I hope my wife will say that about me when I am gone."

"No, he was *literally* a clown."

"Like—"

She slid a flyer in front of me. It said, "Mr. Jiggles will be performing..." with a picture of a real-life clown in makeup, red nose, and all.

Now, I am fairly certain I know what you are thinking here. Clowns = creepy. Whether, in the gutter in the movie *It*, at the circus, notorious serial killers who allegedly were, or at a children's party when you get too close and you notice the mustard stains on the filthy clown suit after he blows a sword out of blue and red balloons for your child. I get it.

But Mr. Jiggles was legit. (I just laughed as I wrote that.)

He was that old school clown with class before clowns became as creepy as the mall Santa.

I looked up and saw Carol waiting for my reaction.

"Cool."

"It's cool, right?" she said hopefully.

"Totally," I said.

"Can we bury him in his clown suit?"

I saw the sheer joy in her eyes. She never thought Leo was

creepy as a clown by that look. She knew the man. She knew he wasn't creepy in any way. She knew the genuine joy he brought to people's lives and she clearly reveled in it too.

"Heck yeah," I said.

"Really?"

"Hell yeah!"

And as the final word of that sentence came out of my mouth, a tidal wave of emotion cascaded from her face, mind, and shoulders and she began to sob uncontrollably.

I reached over and held her hand.

"We had so much joy together, so many laughs. He brought so much humor to so many people's lives."

And you could tell that was true.

So we did it. We prepared his body, placed him in his multicolored, polka-dotted oversized clown suit, clown shoes, and clown makeup, red nose of course, and made Leo into Mr. Jiggles for his final journey.

It was an open casket. And as people approached, they burst out in laughter, almost to a person.

The funeral crowd loved it. There was crying, stories like you wouldn't believe of joy, wonder, and laughter that Leo brought to so many people's lives. It was a memorial service to be remembered forever.

I was reminded how a sense of humor can help us through the troughs in our lives and how people appreciate, and admire, it in another human being. Sure, we all feel differently about clowns. In this case it was different. This was a man who genuinely liked to bring smiles to people's faces. He liked to brighten another human's day. He chose joy. He chose happiness. He chose laughter. He chose smiles.

Carol thanked me. Not any quick, superficial kind of thanks. She gave me a hug, she looked me in the eye, and she genuinely thanked me from the bottom of her soul. I could see how much it meant.

Choose laughter!

LET'S LOOK AT THE SCIENCE

The immune system in our bodies is designed to fight off bad things like microbes, bacteria, and toxins—nasty bugs that will invade your body in an attempt to do it harm. When you are alive, your immune system fights off these harmful bad guys. When you die, for example, you no longer have an immune system to fight off the onslaught of such things. Thus, your body will be eaten by these bacteria and you become a skeleton of bones in just a few weeks' time.

A pleasant visual from the funeral guy. Which is why I believe it is way better to be alive.

In its most rudimentary form, the body works like this: stress hormones, like cortisol, suppress the immune system, which in turn increase the number of blood platelets, which in turn raise your blood pressure. This is why doctors tell you to alleviate stress in your life via exercise, mindfulness, or laughter. Laughter shuts off stress hormones in your body, lowers blood pressure, and increases vascular blood flow and the oxygenation of blood that helps you heal.

I read it on the internet (so we know it's true): "When we laugh, natural killer cells that destroy tumors and viruses increase, as do Gamma-interferon (a disease-fighting protein), T-cells (a major part of the immune response), and B-cells, those antibodies that destroy disease."

In other words, science clearly shows how laughter actually increases the good-guy cells that destroy tumors and viruses.

Bottom line in caveman simplicity: laugh = good.

ROBIN

To me, what stinks about dying is this: you're gone.

Profound, right?

Robin Williams was the greatest comic of my generation. I grew up on *Mork & Mindy*. You could tell very clearly from the first episode you were seeing something special. Then came his legendary stand-up routines, his various movie credits, and his myriad appearances on any number of late-night talk shows. He was a human tour de force. He had that impish grin and squinted eye smile that just drew you in. Even when he segued to more dramatic roles, he had a supremely relatable quality.

Then he kind of faded as movie stars sometimes do, whether they are not being consistently offered the same parts they once were, or they merely decided to take a few years off to be, well, human.

In Robin's case, it seems it was because he had the onset of a disease that affected his mind and motor functions. I don't know the full details, and I suspect we will never know. After all he gave to the public, it is certainly his family's right to be private.

The problem I have is I never felt that he received the due recognition from the world he deserved. We heard of his tragic death, there were some news stories, a CNN special, and he was gone.

Then, I think about the amount of laughter he brought to the human race. How many people saw his movies, shows, TV appearances, and how many people he made laugh through his work in these remarkable films:

- *Good Morning, Vietnam*
- *Mrs. Doubtfire*
- *Jumanji*
- *Cadillac Man*
- *The Birdcage*
- *Aladdin*
- *Patch Adams*
- *Night at the Museum*
- *Happy Feet*
- And the less funny, but equally brilliant *One Hour Photo, Dead Poets Society,* and *Good Will Hunting*

How do we thank a man for the collective belly laugh he brought to the world? The smiles he induced?

I am not as much interested in the trained monkey who is thrown out on stage to do his shtick. I know there has to be an entertainment persona and a private persona. All I am saying is I hope his private persona could look out into our collective universe and say, "I totally frickin' crushed that."

I guess...I guess I simply want to say thank you. Thank you, Robin, for how often you made us all laugh. I want you to know you were "The Man." The best of your generation. And how many of us appreciated all you did for us. The smile you brought to a sad day, the hope you brought through the powerful medium of TV and film, the goodness we felt in that impish smile, the vulnerability, the grace, the dignity, and the insanity you brought to everything you did.

We got robbed from telling you of our adoration for so many more years. Thank you for making us laugh. You frickin' crushed it.

MY DAD

Both of my parents were the children of German immigrants, which makes me immigrant version 2.0. My father had me, his third son, when he was twenty-six. (I had my first son when I was thirty-nine.) My father is one of my best friends, and he makes me laugh like no one else with generally really stupid, immature stuff. Most of the rest of our family can't stand our interplay, but we can't stop.

And here's how it goes down: My dad's mother, Nanie, as she was called, was from Germany. She came over on a boat in 1927. She spoke fluent English by the time I knew her, but what was distinct about her (in addition to her penchant for butter and whipped cream) was the way she said certain words with a heavy German accent.

Over the years, I have come to realize that many of us children of immigrants, or first-generation kids, in America have had the same experience. The children, and certainly the grandchildren, have become fully Americanized, but our parents and/or grandparents have not, but they get by with certain words being "ethnically distinct." Whatever your nationality, it is humorous for the second generation to take these words and bastardize them, or use hyperbole, to make the words even more ridiculous, or humorous, to the rest of your family.

It also reinforces the idea of how our differences are really all the same.

So the words my father and I bastardized in English with a German accent are these:

gloves = glups

lemon = lem

orange = ahh-ing

yellow = jello

And a litany of other clean, semiclean, and filthy words.

When my dad and I go into our bastardized "Nanie diatribe" and begin conversing back and forth in "her" language, it makes us both laugh like no other. We will generally do this around the kitchen, preparing a meal, while everyone else is begging us to stop, culminating in my mom yelling at my dad (not me), despite my willing and overt participation.

But we simply can't stop… and why would we?

MY BOYS AND WIFE

My children also have an uncanny ability to make me laugh, as is the case in most families. It is not usually the belly laugh kind; it is more about what they try to get away with or how they make me remember the same exact shenanigans I tried to pull over on my parents. (Don't they know I was the G.O.A.T. at this game?) Their attempts make me laugh in more of a nostalgic type of way than anything else.

There are also the laughs my wife and I share about our children, generally out of their earshot, or after they have gone to bed. We talk about what they did that made us laugh, their idiosyncrasies, their behavior, things we simply cannot believe.

These are great times of bonding with my wife and laughing about the lives we lead and how insane it is.

One story that particularly encapsulates this for me is our children's inability to eat crusts. While maybe understandable on bread (with an actual crust), they have now extended this insanity to tortillas and bagels. When I explain the edge of a tortilla is EXACTLY THE SAME AS THE BITE YOU JUST TOOK ONE MILLIMETER PRIOR, they just look at me and shake their heads, can't do it.

That shit is insane—funny, but insane. It perfectly describes the type of laughter you receive as a parent.

A second story is perhaps more telling.

Often, I have to admit, I do not feel like a parent to these boys. I feel like my sons are my three best friends and we are simply hanging out together. I think this is bad. Actually, I know this is bad, yet I cannot help it. I am flawed.

I find myself talking to them, not so much as my sons, but as my compadres in this game of life. But there are times when these little men get out of line. They know it and I know it.

Unfortunately, a transgression is usually followed by Dad raising his voice. On this one particular occasion, my youngest son, Mack, was being particularly belligerent, no doubt the result of his multiple cupcake and Honest Kids organic fruit drink consumption from a friend's birthday party hours earlier.

As I raised my voice, Mack saw I was serious and realized he had stepped over the line. He listened to me reiterating the bullet points of his indiscretions over the past twenty minutes that led to my diatribe. As he looked at me, I saw his face visibly softening.

Now I was starting to feel guilty for raising my voice. As I came to a stop to prevent myself from hyperventilating, he simply shook his head at me for a long beat.

Then, he said, "Dad, that's just not the way friends talk to each other."

Case closed.

Being a parent is the greatest joy I have ever been given.

AT YOURSELF

All this talk of incidents and people that make us laugh is superseded by the greatest gift you can give yourself— the ability to laugh—at you.

I believe this will enable you to live a longer, healthier life. Remember the science about killer cells that die when you laugh.

For example, I know I am imperfect as a dad, and that's just fine. I embrace that. I am the softie, clearly the less competent parent. I fart, steal candy from the cupboard, and tell bawdy stories to my sons, which are behaviors a good parent probably should not do.

Boys, I will pay the therapy bills.

However, I believe it shows my sons that adults are human too. I figure if I set the bar low enough, there will be tons of victories in life, and who doesn't like victories?

When Angie and I were raising babies, there was a book called *Battle Hymn of the Tiger Mother* by Amy Chua (2011). Dude, that woman had it locked down. It talked about extreme discipline and raising your child to be a high achiever and excel at everything. Whether you believed the author was writing a self-mocking portrayal of her own life or a how-not-to indictment on Western parenting is up to you. Rock solid book, smart woman.

We have a friend who is a tiger mom, a super high achiever, raising a family of high achievers. It is amazing to witness their activities, scheduling, and overall academic prowess, so perfectly crafted as if in a human genome laboratory: rapid learner programs, fencing (easier way in to Stanford), classical piano, Mandarin lessons, summer academic hiking camps in Gstaad, how to build a rocket ship with sippy straws. It is awe-inspiring to witness from my imperfect distance.

Now, I want the best for my kids, and I am as guilty as the next guy of trying to do a little extra. For example, I played classical music when our children were infants so they would fall asleep to Mozart and Beethoven in the comforts of their crib; I read somewhere it made the neurons and protons in their brains formulate better to improve their intelligence.

Yeah, it didn't.

Take it from this panda dad (the soft and squishy kind), my child may not graduate summa cum laude from Wharton, but he will know how much his dad loves him. And I'll take that any day of the week.

If your failures, your idiosyncrasies, the situations or predicaments you are in are able to be laughed at, you rebound quicker from your problems. Some people are better at this than others. I would just say, if we could all learn to be less harsh on ourselves, and see the humor in being human, I think we could solve more of the ills of the world than we realize.

The ability to laugh at ourselves gives us the perspective needed to bounce back from seeming defeat. I wish I could tell this to my younger self. When you are young, everything seems so grave, so heightened, so make-or-break. This is simply not the case; it is never the case. There is always another boy or girl, always another school or job, always another environment in which you will thrive.

Know that—always! Find the funny in being human. I guarantee good things will happen from there.

―――――――

IN SUM

The science about laughter is there; it is evident. The more you laugh, the healthier you will be. What is unscientific is that it does not matter how you laugh, but simply that you do it for your well-being. Special people, like Mr. Jiggles and Robin Williams, have been placed on this earth to make others laugh. Find them, find the people, the situations that make you laugh and repeat, repeat, and repeat again.

But the greatest gift is the ability to laugh at yourself; never fail to see the humor in your own actions. This will give you the perspective to realize that circumstances in life can't possibly always go our way.

Laugh, people, just laugh.

THE REMINDERS

Laughter truly is our best medicine.

Try to laugh as much as possible.

Be with those who make you laugh.

Laugh at yourself.

---

13 Enjoy Food

"Oh, and one last thing. I have a letter for you," I told the woman who was already exhausted from making funeral arrangements for her father.

She looked at me oddly.

"It's from your dad."

She looked up at me as if to say, really, dude?

She opened the sealed letter in front of me. She paused for a moment to read it. I simply sat there and watched her. She began to smile and tear up. She took a deep breath. "Did you do this?"

"No, ma'am," I said. "The letter was taped to his pre-need file."

Short break here. I need to explain. A pre-need in the funeral world is when someone arranges for and usually pays for their funeral prior to it happening, usually a long time before. The proceeds are held in the third-party trust or insurance company, and the funeral home simply sends the third party a death certificate when the person dies, and the funds are released to the funeral home. The funds are held by a third party to ensure that the funeral proceeds are certain to be available when the person dies. Now you know.

I asked, "What's it say?"

She handed me the letter and it went something like this:

Hey, monkey. I love you.

Thank you for all you've done to make life so great.

As you already know, my favorite times were when we were all together celebrating any number of family occasions or holidays. Sitting at Prego, everyone eating their favorite meals, even if it was buttered noodles.

This was where I was happiest. In the middle of it all, sitting back in my chair and just…watching.

My bliss.

I hope you keep this up when I am gone.

After my funeral, I have paid for everyone to go to Prego again.

Say nice things about me. I have loved you all.

I looked back at her. Now I started tearing up. "I have those places with my family too."

She sat there crying and nodding, "It's so him. It's who he was."

Food does that for people, for families.

BOURDAIN

Anthony Bourdain died.

I loved his show (*Anthony Bourdain: Parts Unknown* on CNN). He traveled to exotic places and ate the finest foods, the street food, and the food in people's homes. It was exhilarating to watch him share a meal and then probe deeper into the cultures, the politics, and the heartbeat of the people of the city or country he was in. He seemed so learned, but not in any pretentious way. I guess he had this chef/Everyman quality that made me feel like he was one of us.

My admiration for him stemmed from the fact that he was what true New Yorkers would agree was a real New Yorker at heart. I am from Westchester (I know real New Yorkers think that is upstate), and I knew many people like him. I heard he grew up in the suburbs of Jersey and had a nice childhood, like I did.

It seems he had a wanderlust that I never had, but maybe that is what made me like him even more. He would travel the world over and eat all these exotic dishes in faraway locales, and I could simply be a voyeur on his journey from the comforts of my L.L. Bean goose down comforter and My Pillow pillows.

His enjoyment of both food and drink were palpable, but he seemed, more so, to have a preternatural curiosity to discover what made the people of the country, or locale, tick. He was so much more than a foodie to me. It seemed he had an inherent desire to comprehend the places he visited, especially in countries whose heritage was so many generations older than our own.

I know nothing about the man. But I do know he felt if we all sat down and had a meal and a few drinks together, maybe we could start to see some of the commonalities in all of us as humans, no matter the location of our piece of earth on the globe. And, with that, I wholeheartedly agree.

As a true fan, I am sorry for the pain he must have had. I am sorry we couldn't have helped him. But I am grateful for what he brought to our bedrooms at night. I enjoyed watching him, empathizing with people of different cultures, and learning.

God bless you, Tony, although I am fairly certain you didn't believe in Him. God bless you and I hope to have a pastrami sandwich together when it's all over.

THE HOUSE OF PAIN

I have always been a sucker for a Chinese buffet. The idea of being able to eat a little, or a lot, of everything on the menu has always been right in my wheelhouse. Ming Garden, in Chestnut Hill, Massachusetts, was a glorious buffet in college; Oriental Luau in Thornwood, New York, was an excellent one growing up; and when I was in law school, we found one thirty minutes away in the town of Montpelier, famously the home of the Ben & Jerry's ice cream factory. It was a magnificent place.

I am truly uncertain of how we came to find this restaurant, probably a recommendation of a fellow student, but we had about five guys in our crew who liked to eat. One in particular was of Chinese descent, Baldwin Chin. Baldwin was a thick-necked guy from Houston who spoke with a Texas twang. He was an exceptionally happy guy who liked to join in whenever food was mentioned.

So picture this.

Middle of Vermont, large Chinese guy with Texas twang rolling into a Chinese buffet in the state's capital. The only thing that could make it more bizarre was the half-insane owner of the restaurant, and the House of Pain (as we would call it because that's how we felt after overeating there) had such a man. He was straight out of a Soderbergh movie: toupee, rail thin, perennial smile, and an overly happy, close talker. You can probably imagine his joy when we rolled in with Baldwin.

This guy reacted as if he had seen the second coming of Lao Tzu. He would run up to Baldwin, grab his arm, and simply look him up and down for a long beat before saying: "You China man?"

Baldwin would respectfully reply, "Yes, sir." Then awkwardly look over at the rest of us as if to say what the—

More looks up and down, then looks over at us, then back to Baldwin.

"You too big to be China man."

We all burst out laughing.

"You way too big to be China man."

Now, mind you, Baldwin was big, but not fat. He was just a solid dude. But scrutiny wouldn't stop. The owner just looked at B and marveled, generally, to the point of making us all more uncomfortable than eating his oyster egg foo yong. He was a gentle soul who loved B and held a special place in all of our hearts. He loved us because our group would grow and grow as people back at law school started to hear our stories. I remember a few women coming up to me back at school saying, "We went up there and that food was disgusting."

I simply looked at them and said, "I know."

That's the funny thing about food; sometimes it's never about the food.

FAMILY DINNERS

Family dinners are the quintessential times when most of us think about enjoying food. Families share food with each other—occasions that often preserve traditions, cultures, and relationships that are important to each one of us. Mealtime is a perfect way to pass on the history of us all to the younger generations.

I would argue that this is an integral, if not seminal, part of family and preservation of who we are as a people—recognizing our uniqueness. I encourage us all to dig deep and never let these times go by the wayside. Our traditions are us; they are vital to our families' preservation. Teach, learn, pass on.

In my own life, my mom was an amazing cook. She was trained by her mother, my Oma, and that woman would have a warm meal ready for you every night. You'd come home from practice and the smells would be intoxicating. She often speaks of the joy I brought to her day because I would always walk in the front door and shout, "What's for dinner?" And she wouldn't just make standard stuff. She made stuffed flank steak, sweet and sour pork, different dishes that took time. Looking back on it, I was one lucky kid. I remember really enjoying our meals almost every night and my mom smiling as we ate.

I came to learn that food was another way my mother showed us love. She was always affectionate and tucked us all in, but, as a homemaker, she was showing us her love through her food.

We had a large family (Dad had a brother and twin sisters),

and I had seven cousins who got together every Christmas Eve, Thanksgiving, and Easter for about fifteen years straight. I remember the open-face sandwiches on Christmas Eve at Aunt Joan's in Nyack where we would always have to leave by 10:00 p.m. to get to midnight Mass back home. Thanksgivings and Easters were rotated among our house, my aunt's, and my grandmother's where we would always enjoy a turkey with the traditional fixings; all of those women were amazing cooks.

In later years, we'd go to the Casa Hofbrau, a local joint in Emerson, New Jersey, where we feasted on stuffed clams (at least I think they were clams) and Shirley Temples. The food was always a focal point that acted as an excuse to get together. I remember how much I enjoyed being with my cousins—some older, some younger.

For me, it was what family was all about.

Death, drama, and bad blood have all precluded those times from happening again. Family stuff has intervened. The fighting— it's such a waste. I miss those times we had breaking bread with our extended family.

IN SUM

Look, you are either a foodie or you're not. Most people I know like food. The thing about food for me is it locks in memories in time with friends or family; the ceremonious breaking of bread enables us all to recollect people and moments, whether holidays with family, nights out with friends, or study breaks from the rigors of school to laugh at the real world. I have loved food since I was a small child. For me, sharing food offers us all a commonality of joy from where to start the conversation.

I think we probably all take for granted these times of sharing a meal and talking around a table with one another. And I know Anthony Bourdain was right: Sharing food with one another would solve a lot of the world's ills. He knew if we sat down, had a meal together, and started drinking and talking, we could learn more about each other and more clearly see our common ground. I know there is way more common ground than any of us realize.

For me, there is something quite intimate about food and having a meal together. Food, in many ways, is an expression of love, of caring, of sharing, of kindness. It is saying I prepared this for you and please enjoy. It's what moms, dads, grandmas, and grandpas do the world over. They are sharing part of themselves, their history, their culture, and their love.

Enjoy food. It's an expression of love. Serve it and eat it with that in mind and it might change a few things in our world.

THE REMINDERS

Food is adventure and memories.

---

*Bourdain was right, breaking bread together
would solve a lot of the ills of the world.*

---

*Food enables us to recollect special moments
in time with those we love.*

Food is an expression of love made by the right person.

You can always find something at a Chinese food buffet.

14 Sweat, Fiber, and Water

One of the most nerve-racking parts of owning a funeral home is how a body looks after being embalmed. Embalming is the process of draining blood from the veins and pumping tinted fluid back into them with the goal of making the person simply look as if they are sleeping when they are viewed by family and friends.

That is the goal.

Invariably, people are not good candidates for embalming (like with victims of heart disease, hardening of the arteries, or stroke), but their loved ones still want to view them. We always ask families to bring in a picture of their loved one, so we can get an idea of how they should appear: their hairstyle, their makeup, any noteworthy items like wearing glasses regularly. Almost always, the photos we are provided are from a time when the decedent was healthy, vital, and thriving—like at a trattoria on Lake Como thirty years prior.

You are starting to understand the challenge, right?

This image from the past, coupled with people living an unhealthy lifestyle as they age and the cause of their death, all further complicate matters. If a family looks at you and wonders why "Grandpa doesn't look like the photo I gave you," it is hard not to look them back in the eye and say, "Because he probably didn't eat right or exercise in the last forty years"—even if that's what you might be thinking.

Conversely, I have been in the exact opposite situations—for example, where a woman had a massive brain hemorrhage and the coroner had to do an autopsy to ascertain the cause of death. In doing so, the coroner had to make an incision around the scalp, which is usually done in a very crude manner. Not something a family needs to witness.

In this particular instance, the family wisely chose to have a closed casket.

But at the church, one of the nieces wanted to see her aunt one last time. The family said it was okay.

The funeral home is saying WTF? Since we were told no one would see her, we did not prepare the body for viewing. Generally speaking, funeral homes do not like last-minute surprises—as you could imagine.

In this case, the niece peeked inside the casket and thought her aunt looked amazing. You simply never know.

STRAIGHT TALK

Okay. Now the funeral guy's guide to healthy living.

How am I qualified?

Fitness gurus think they know what will make you live longer. I have seen what will kill you. You choose which one of us to believe.

In my fourteen years of owning a funeral home, I rarely buried a super fit person who hadn't died on a motorcycle.

Period.

You gotta sweat. If you want to live long, you gotta sweat. America needs to cut the Fitbit shit and stop being fascinated with how many steps you took. It ain't that impressive.

"Hey, look, I lifted my arm and took a dump too." Crushin' it!

Take that Fitbit and jam it right back up the keister of corporate America.

Look, it's great to exercise and go for walks, stretch, count your steps, whatever, as long as you're moving, but if you don't sweat, it doesn't truly work. I am as guilty of this as the next guy. I love to take walks in the morning to clear my brain. It's awesome, but it doesn't work like sweating. And your sweating does not have to be for too long (based on no sound medical testimony but my own), I think anything over twenty-five minutes of actual sweating, and you are good to go. Do it three to five times a week and make sure you're having sex too (at least that's what I tell my wife).

"Get off me!" Angie says.

"It's for my health!"

Second, hydrate your body with water. It is the simplest thing on earth and has profound effects on the inner workings of your plumbing and the appearance (via your skin) you will portray to the world. The problem is you will have to pee a lot more. A small sacrifice for staying healthy.

The elderly have a real concern about peeing all the time because they don't want to keep getting up and down and going to the bathroom. To them, these movements to and from the bathroom

LIFE IN 20 LESSONS

are all potential accident opportunities for slipping, falling, and breaking a hip. I get it, but this has to happen. Dehydration in the elderly is a massive health issue.

Please hydrate. Everyone!

Third, you need to lift if you don't want your muscles to atrophy. If muscles aren't pushed, you endanger your endoskeleton. The endoskeleton goes, and you are in the hospital or rehab. Nothing against hospitals or rehab, but...

Last, stay away from sugar. It is the antichrist to our bodies. No exceptions! (I write this to you while eating a Snickers bar; I am simply not that good.)

So, you must sweat, hydrate, lift, no sugar—and have sex.

THE STORY OF POOP

I love poop.

I love everything about it. It's fun to talk about, look at, and smells horrible. I have three sons and it dominates our lives. It comes in all shapes, sizes, and consistencies. Once I even found what appeared to be a raisin on the floor.

That's...not...A RAISIN!

My wife is a saint.

I'm a dad who changed diapers too. You see things when you change diapers that humble you. You see what these little humans are capable of. It becomes a form of early respect, like, dang, little man, that's impressive. How many of you haven't run to your spouse, arms outstretched with a full diaper, and said, "Look at this!"

"What did you feed this child? Organic beets and chipped beef?"

Anyone?

No one in my family seems to love poop as much as I do. In fact, I can distinctly remember my mom getting angry at me when I would speak about it, generally at the kitchen table. That all changed the day Oprah did a story about poop. Yup, the Big O did an entire episode about it with Dr. Oz.

Finally, I thought, poop had slid its way back into the American lexicon and become conversational. You know, if Oprah talks about it—

In the episode, she and Dr. Oz talked about the three characteristics you should look for in your poop: sound as it hits the water (should be "like an Acapulco cliff diver"), color, and shape (it should be an S, banana, or have a curve to it. And, no, you should not lift yourself off the bowl in an attempt to create these shapes). The episode was truly fascinating to me as a funeral guy, because I couldn't agree more. The flow of effluent through your personal plumbing system is vital to a long life. It means things are working correctly inside your body.

And the key to this flow in my opinion is fiber! Natural is always better, but for busy lives, Metamucil works.

At the time of this writing, I have no personal stock in Procter & Gamble (P&G), Metamucil's parent company. I simply believe if you all took Metamucil (the powder, not the pills) for two weeks straight, religiously, it would change your lives and you would call me and ask me to be your personal, professional, and spiritual caca messiah.

My brother told me about this miracle powder, and it gave me a personal renaissance in the Era of Poop Enlightenment.

Metamucil, or psyllium husk, is a shortcut for people with busy lives, or for those who do not eat correctly, to get a quick dose of fiber in their diet. It would be much better to get your fiber organically by eating fruits, vegetables, and legumes, but that is not always possible with our overly busy lives.

Try Metamucil for two weeks straight and call me; I'll probably be their spokesman by then.

The other pearl I am going to give you is the age-old adage we have all heard a million times: "An apple a day keeps the doctor away."

Why? Because it works.

It was advice given when people didn't have Metamucil. Some old-timer didn't want the town crier to have to scream about poop up and down the cobblestone streets of ye merry ol' England, but he knew all about it. He figured, if I simply tell them to eat an apple a day, it will be the best thing for them, and I won't have to explain the whole poop thing and maybe face the queen's guillotine for talking about such filthy topics. That guy (or gal) who came up with the saying was a medieval precursor to Dr. Oz.

Now, to do fiber a solid, so to speak, you should really get the natural stuff. And this is where we start thinking about food as medicine. Anything grown in nature that is green, orange, red, or purple is best:

- Green: I personally think broccoli is the super food of the world. Think about it. When you eat broccoli, it's as if that cruciferous-ness (I know that is not a word, yet it is a completely accurate and perfect nonword) pulls "things" through your colon. Pure magic!

- Orange: Carrots, pumpkin, or sweet potatoes—throw a little olive oil on them and roast at 425 degrees for thirty minutes and your kids will think they are eating candy.
- Red: Tomatoes any way you can get them is good, especially for dudes.
- Purple: Cabbage and beets, cut them up and put dressing on them if you have to make it taste better (two more super foods).

Finally, legumes or beans. Eat as many as you want, they are cheap, easy to prepare, go with anything, and you will feel lighter and never be hungry. Fiber!

So, you see, sweat, hydration, poop, and food as medicine are all interrelated. If you sweat, hydrate, and eat right, it makes the poop look right.

And we all want good-looking poop.

IN SUM

It is no coincidence this chapter on sweat, fiber, and water follows a chapter about how to enjoy food because, like Newton's third law said, "With every action there is an equal and opposite reaction." And merely encouraging people to exercise is really not enough for me because I firmly believe you need to truly sweat when you work out, and, in this funeral guy's eyes, add fiber and water as the most salient keys to your longevity in this world. With these three (and their natural offshoots), I believe there will be proper flow through your body, and, like the plumbing in your house, we all need proper flow.

I'm a funeral guy, trust me. I see the ravages of time and lack of exercise, water, and fiber. You can trust the fitness gurus' theories or the funeral guy's facts. Your call.

THE REMINDERS

There are not a ton of dead fit people.

Sweat, actually sweat, when you exercise.

Sex, yes (and tell Angie too).

Pump some iron with resistance training.

Hydrate with water.

Analyze your poop.

Eat colors grown in nature (green, orange, red, purple).

---

15 Stop Worrying about Money

Bruce was my parents' neighbor. He lived across the street with his wife and five children, all under twelve years of age when my parents moved in. I was back and forth at college and law school, so I simply knew Bruce in passing.

In the winters at my parents' house, it was beautiful, idyllic really. Their property overlooked a pond that would freeze over. People from around the neighborhood would come over and either skate, run around, or play hockey. It was a real slice-of-life gathering place, and my parents loved watching the kids play and going out to chat with their neighbors.

If I were home, invariably, I would go out and chat with Bruce. He was a real man's man, a bond trader on Wall Street, generally had a drink in his hand and always a smile on his face. He loved life, and he was clearly having fun living it with his family, and it showed.

On our few talks, he always asked about my life, offered words of encouragement, and told me how he admired my folks. He was easy to like. A couple of evenings when my parents were away, he saw some shenanigans over at our house in the wee hours of the morning (suspected streakers and the like), which he let me know he saw, but never shared with my folks.

He was crazy cool.

I played ball with guys like Bruce. They rode the train into the city from Westchester every day, worked their asses off, and got back on the train to get ready for the next day. These guys were nails in my eyes because that is a grind, in all kinds of weather, no matter how much money you are making. Respect.

I got a call from my mother a few days after 9/11 when the Towers were struck.

She said Bruce called his wife and said, "I'm not going to make it out this time." (Bruce had survived the previous fire at the World Trade Center.) He did not survive. I thought of his wife and children. Knowing someone always brings such tragic events closer.

So why tell you this story of my parents' neighbor?

Because Bruce went to work that day to simply provide for his family, put in a few more years, then kick it some place and fish. His children never got to see their dad grow old with them and be at their graduations, weddings—you know, the good stuff.

I want us all to stop worrying about money because life is random. Indiscriminate. Unpredictable.

Bruce just went to work that day. He just went to work.

STOP WORRYING ABOUT MONEY

BOGLEHEAD

Money doesn't buy happiness. True.

Yet, we need money to live. Granted.

We have to save for retirement. Yes.

But if you are conservative and disciplined, you can do it.

Look, I'm a Boglehead at heart. I believe in everything the late John Bogle, the founder of the Vanguard Group, believed in: low-cost, index fund investing. Bogle simply believed we should not have to pay an advisor, or fund, or fees for something that is a lot less complicated than everyone tries to make it. He was revolutionary in his thinking and probably angered a great many people on Wall Street in doing so when he first started.

While I did not know him at all, I suspect he didn't care what others said about him. He brought index investing to Main Street and beyond, simplifying a seemingly confusing process. I admire him because he tapped right into my pauper mentality, the grand cheapskate inside of me shouting at every turn: I want a deal.

And Bogle always had the altruism of helping the masses on his side, which was his true genius because he parlayed that into a billion-dollar fortune, right?

Do we care? I don't, but I suspect millions of financial advisors got out of that vocation when, and if, they saw the Vanguard tsunami approaching.

Thank you, Mr. Bogle, for making investing easier for us all.

EVERY PROFESSIONAL ATHLETE ON THE PLANET

I am a junkie for ESPN's *30 for 30*, *E:60*, or any show using the combination of sports, heart, tragedy, and triumph. The stories of money loss and embezzlement are among the most tragic to me.

Now, I am sending out a plea to athletes all over the world: Please find me and I will help you.

I am not a financial advisor, but I am fairly certain you do not need one. Do not listen to your agent, your league, your momma, or your homeboy who took college prep finance courses at your local community college or online. Separate yourself from everyone you know and find me. I will show you how to place everything in your name only, no powers of attorney, and you will understand what you are investing in (like a few of Mr. Bogle's funds); no one will be responsible for your money, but you. No one!

End of story.

We will assume your career will end tomorrow, and we will attempt to make your money last a lifetime based on historical (past) returns, all the while clearly understanding there are no absolute certainties in the stock market; all we have is the past returns (history) to look at.

No one has a crystal ball, no matter what they tell you.

And, most importantly, you will understand the tax ramifications of everything you do.

If you are extremely lucky, you can help those closest to you, but you must take care of you and your future first. It will not be popular among any of your inner circle. People will try to make you feel guilty for forgetting about your roots, but it will be the best thing for you and your future. Please see any of the numbers of athletes who have lost everything in investments that I am certain made sense to someone, at some time. Out of respect, I will not list them, but they are well documented on the internet.

Slow and steady wins the race—always.

And, it gets easier.

When talk of investing arises, I always direct everyone who will listen to *Lazy Portfolios* (www.marketwatch.com/lazyport-folio). Now, I have many friends who are financial advisors, and they are good men and women, but, for me, this encapsulates how I feel about Wall Street. At the time of this writing (January 5, 2019), the S&P 500 (one of the most popular averages advisors compare themselves to) returned the best ten-, five-, three-, and one-year annualized returns, even as compared to these simple portfolios. That sounds reasonable, and I think Mr. Bogle would smile about that.

What I find most interesting is the second-best performer over that exact same time period was what *Lazy Portfolios* calls the "Second Grader's Starter" portfolio: "Kevin's an eight-year-old second grader who started with a gift from grandma and a few hints from his father. This is a very simple portfolio of three no-load index funds for a new investor with a little money" (www.marketwatch.com/lazyportfolio/portfolio/second-grader-starter).

What I find equally interesting is this portfolio beat a slew of professionally managed portfolios with great financial minds investing their money. The simple meaning is we all overcomplicate things, including, and especially, investing our own money.

A few poignant observations—

1. If you are working your ass off to make money and are able to save enough to invest, why are you giving it to someone else to place somewhere? Because it feels better? Less pressure? Educate yourself and take ownership of your hard-earned money.

2. Do not listen to anyone who has a quick money scheme or something too good to be true. The world is littered with hucksters in $50 and $5,000 suits. And don't be hard on yourself, we have all been there; we have all been taken by the allure of quick money. For example, my former girlfriend, her brother, and I played three-card monte in NYC and lost $60 in a nanosecond. We were stupid, naive kids from the 'burbs, fresh meat to these con artists with collapsible, cardboard tables. I just wished it happened to all of us at nineteen years old with $60 instead of at sixty years old with our life savings. If you invest with someone who promises you pie-in-the-sky returns, then you are the idiot who believed you could beat the system, or you saw easy money. Money is made slowly over long periods of time. Put it somewhere safe and forget about it; stop reading and believing the hype. Educate yourself and make smart decisions.

3. Here it is simply: When you take in two bucks, don't spend three, and always look for the best deal.

Done.

COMPOUNDING

The greatest lesson my father and grandfather ever taught me was about the power of compounding. If you have a moment, please show your child this website called Money Chimp (www.money-chimp.com/calculator/compound_interest_calculator.htm).

Then, place the numbers in bold on the right in the corresponding boxes:

Current principal place **$10,000**

Annual addition **$7,400**

Years to grow....................................... **40**

Interest rate **5%**

Compound interest .... **1** time(s) annually

Then, hit the "Calculate" box with your mouse. The "Future Value" should read:

$1,009,014

This means if you start with $10,000 in savings and put $7,400 away each year (or $616.67 per month) from twenty-five years of age until you retire at sixty-five, you will be a millionaire. And this is figured at a very modest 5% return on your money. Your original $10,000 plus the $296,000 you contributed over that forty-year period became $1,009,014.

So, if I invest $306,000, I will make $1,009,014.

Who wouldn't do that deal?

Now, granted, not everyone can put away $7,400 each year nor may everyone need a million dollars in retirement, but, hopefully, you can clearly see the point of my exercise.

And it gets even crazier.

And please don't trust me, I have no horse in this race; simply check the data at Business Insider (www.businessinsider.com/30-year-sp-500-returns-impressive-2016-5). This article talks about the S&P 500 average returns over three thirty-year periods:

1926–1956: +10.77%
1956–1986: +9.63%
1986–2016: +9.99%

If we take the worst of those thirty-year period averages (9.63%) and plug it into our equation, watch what happens:

Current principal place **$10,000**
Annual addition **$7,400**
Years to grow... **40**
Interest rate **9.63%**
Compound interest .... **1** time(s) annually

Then, hit "Calculate" box with your mouse. The "Future Value" should read:

$ 3,643,333

If I invest $306,000, I will receive $3,643,333.

Don't overthink retirement. Your money will compound for you. That is the simple power of compounding.

The problem humans have is we are emotional with our money. When the stock market goes down, we pull our money out; when it goes up, we invest more. That is what I mean when I say we are emotional with our money. This is exactly the wrong tactic. We need to take the emotion out of our finances. It is counterintuitive, it feels wrong, but it is correct.

The money is made when markets are down. Like Warren Buffett has always said, "Be a buyer when things are bad." And if you can't do that, at least leave your money alone. History shows us that markets always, *always*, come back stronger. If you can't stomach that, then keep your money under your mattress.

It's so darn easy.

***

IN SUM

So much is made about making enough money to retire and being able to live comfortably as we age; yet no one knows a particular formula, nor do any of us spend or behave the same way with money. Talk of this seems to dominate every business and news site out there. I believe many of us tend to overcomplicate finances or stick our proverbial heads in the sand when it comes to money.

The irony is that it is much simpler than we think with all of the various investment vehicles readily available to us and with the true star of the money world, the power of compounding. The sooner we recognize that money is not that complicated, we should similarly realize there are no guarantees we will get to enjoy the fruits of our retirement labor. Remember, Bruce just went to work that day on September, the eleventh, 2001. One day at a time, as the saying goes.

THE REMINDERS

Do not worry about money, we have no idea what tomorrow brings.

Becoming a millionaire is not that difficult, if that's even important to you.

Life is indiscriminate. Love, above all, love.

Start today.

---

16 Have Faith or Spirituality

The greatest part of my day is when I tuck my children in at night; each of my sons requests it.

"Dad, can you snuggle me?"

How do you say no to that?

For me, these quiet moments alone with each of my sons are so special. They are tired after a long day, as am I, and we just lie there and talk. Sometimes it is just nonsense; sometimes there are very pointed questions; and sometimes there are epic, earth-shattering conversations I'm not quite ready for like when my nine-year-old son Brock asked me: "What happens when you die, Dad?"

Have you ever tried to explain this to your child? My answer was based on my belief system.

I said, "You go to heaven and you are with the ones you love for all of eternity."

"What's eternity?"

"Forever and ever, Brock."

"So you will see your grandpa who died?"

"Yes, I will see Opa. He will be waiting there for me."

"So you will be waiting for me when I die?"

A deep, hard swallow and a long beat. "Yes, Boo, I will be waiting."

Brock thought for a minute. There was total quiet. I knew there had to be more.

"How will you find me?"

"God will lead me to you."

"Are you sure? 'Cause it sounds like a pretty big place, and I don't want to get lost up there."

"I will be waiting for you with open arms, and we will be with each other for ever and ever."

I looked into Brock's eyes. In that one singular moment, I may have never felt closer to another human being than that—the eye connection.

He kept staring at me. He now realized that life is temporary. That I will not be here forever. His eyes filled with tears. And seeing that, my eyes welled up too. I pulled him closer and we embraced.

"I will find you," I whispered.

I could feel a calmness in his body. I could feel the love of his embrace and how much this child loved every fiber of my being.

After a long time, I kissed his cheek, and I said, "That won't be for a long time so let's make sure we love each other every day." That's what you tell a child to show them confidence and keep their mind from spinning, even when you're not sure as an adult.

He smiled and said, "I love you, Daddy. I love you a lot." Something he says each and every night to me, as if to signify he feels more than just love for me. Love, plus even more.

I went to bed, told my wife the story, and cried. I cried a thousand more tears. It was one of the most intimate conversations I had ever had with another human being because it was so honest and real. That's why I love being a dad.

It was epic and my faith and spirituality were my guide.

PASTOR CARY

I have said many times over, owning a funeral home was the greatest gift this world has given me. In my place as the owner, I would be quite active in my local community to make myself known.

In doing so, I have met many fascinating people, but perhaps no one with whom I had a closer connection to than the pastor of a small congregation in town. He was brought in from Alabama during a pastor search to help attract younger families to their aging church population. You see, churches are businesses too.

We met a few times at various functions and slowly became friends. One day, I asked him to go to lunch for no other reason than to get to know him better. From that moment on, we struck a multiple-year friendship. He had two sons, I had three; he loved sports and family, I did too.

He seemed to genuinely care about me and wondered why a guy like me would not bring his family to church after having been raised in a church my whole life. He clearly wanted my family as parishioners. He wanted me to know God, and he even went so far as to gift me a Bible. He was goodness through and through, and he truly believed in the word of the Lord, like few I have ever met in my life. He was in no way pious, judgmental, or reprimanding. In fact, it almost seemed as if he would get a good laugh at me and think to himself, "Spare him, Lord. He will understand one day."

I found myself looking forward to our lunches. We both enjoyed food and would talk about nothing in particular and always had fun doing it. We just enjoyed each other's company.

At one of our lunches, I remember our dialogue went like this:

"So do you believe in God, Chris?"

"I do."

"Then, what's the problem?"

A long beat as I stared down at my shredded chicken tacos covered in a light picante.

"It's just…I just…," I struggled to say.

Another beat. I looked up at him. I looked him right in the eye: "How do I know it's God I'm talking to and not just a voice in my head?"

Now, I am thinking, being a man of the cloth, of course, he's going to say it's God. The other choice would be to let me know it's just a voice in my head, and maybe it's time to check myself in. But, being a pastor, he did the right thing. He leaned over, all dramatic, and said, "It's Him!"

And now I got all dramatic, too, glaring back at him: "But why me? Why am I so special?"

Never missing a beat he replied, "You're not."

Sobering religious shot across the bow. "He talks to everyone."

Well, if that ain't a kick in the religious crotch. My look of confusion registered like a lightning bolt to his eyes.

"The voice in your head is Him. He guides us all."

So the cynic in all of us would say it's just a pastor telling me what I want to hear. And maybe that's just where your faith, or spirituality, rubber meets the proverbial religious road. Do you want to believe? Or do you want to just think it's you?

No correct answer.

And I may be a little crazier than most because I hear two distinct voices: one me and one Him.

So, Pastor convinced me I was talking to God that day, and I have to say that gave me a great deal of solace knowing I had a little one-on-one time with the Big Fella, sort of like I had his number if, and when, I needed him.

Thank you, Pastor Cary. I miss you.

PASTOR PEARSON

As I mentioned, I grew up a Lutheran and went to church every Sunday for the first eighteen years of my life. We had one of the greatest men I have ever known, John Pearson, as our pastor. He was a dynamic preacher and a kind, loving, and thoughtful man. He taught us all about "random acts of kindness," "warm fuzzies and cold pricklies," the power of music, butterfly releases in the middle of church, and, in general, a joie de vivre that made his sermons a time to pay attention. He was the reason people came to church. His holiday services were beyond inspiring, and he sang with the gusto of ten men.

Looking back, I think how lucky I was to be in his church.

He was also a close family friend, and I experienced his love, whether Pastor was dropping off a bag of donuts on a Sunday morning for no reason at all or sitting in front of a fireplace telling us war stories of his time in WWII.

The greatness of this man cannot be understated. He loved to preach the word of the Lord. You could clearly see the Lord working through him. But he was able to place it aside and be human, not sanctimonious in any way, shape, or form, as if he could stop being a preacher now and again.

I wish you could have known this man. He was simply a great man. His heart gave out at a young age, leaving us all devoutly devastated. A day that will live in infamy in Emanuel's collective conscious.

Till we meet again, my friend. I loved you and Mrs. P more than you could ever know.

See, for me, my childhood Lutheranism turned into Judaism-lite through a great girlfriend and many amazing college friends, which turned into a deeper spirituality during my writing years, which then turned into a vocation that created in me an unwavering belief in a Higher Power without ever going to church. I have seen too many amazing occurrences, heard too many stories of survivals and miracles, seen too many happenings of utter beauty for there not to be a Higher Power, that I happen to call God.

My way is not the right way. It is simply the way that works for me. I respect whatever people choose to believe in. But, damn, there has God-a-be more than this for all of us, right?

IN SUM

Formalized religion is not for everyone, and, it seems, at least in our country, for better or worse, people are shying away from it. Maybe because religion mistakenly functions as a great divider, when it should be one of our greatest unifiers. And perhaps it's because there always seems to be the qualifier that you are not truly one of us unless you believe "our" way; in my opinion, that's the greatest flaw among religions.

If your Higher Power is truly this amazing being, wouldn't They love all of us no matter what we believed in? Isn't that what Higher Powers would say? Come one, come all? I believe there is a Higher Power at the center of all this. I believe He (or She) would welcome all of us, all religions, all nonbelievers, everyone, no line drawing.

Look, most of us believe in something. I am not here to change that. I am simply here to say I believe in something. It gives me hope. It gives my children peace and solace and helps me think about those whom I have lost but will see again. Belief gets me through my day. I have seen a lot. I have seen a lot by being in the funeral business. I believe in miracles, and I believe in an afterlife. For me, it's just God-a-be. But you decide for you.

Whomever, bless you.

THE REMINDERS

Believe as you wish, just respect it all.

———

Be comforted by what belief brings to its believer.

———

Children help us see the world more clearly.

———

Think of how much lighter our world would be if we believed there was a better place hereafter.

———

17 Embrace the Elderly

The smell is the first thing that hits you.

It is not foul. It is not fresh. It is somewhere on the lower end of the spectrum in between the industrial clean of a janitor's closet in the school gym mixed with... with...with something else that is not quite right. And it's thick. Thicker than normal air. Not right, un-right in terms of breathing.

The hallway is nondescript. Laminate flooring for easy cleanup. An overworked and underpaid nurse sits looking harried at the hub where four hallways meet. The hallways are lined with elderly men and women. Some hunched over in wheelchairs in awkward positions asleep, some drooling on themselves, some eating, some staring off into the clouds of another world, and one or two smiling, trying to make eye contact with me as if to say hello, come talk to me.

It is a devastating sight to witness. This is elder care in America. And this is a nice facility, "standard" by classification to those in the know.

When I ask the nurse what's going on, she never makes eye contact and explains this is exercise time.

No sweatin' to the oldies here.

To stand at the nursing station and look down the four hallways lined with people was one of the most remarkably tragic moments of my funeral life. Who cares about all these people? These are someone's mother or father, sister or brother, aunt or uncle. These people are someone.

Many of us are insulated from having to witness this parade: the result of our busy lives or healthy parents, or lack of desire to see what this is all about.

My heart hurts. My heart hurts, not for the gentleman I am here to pick up on this particular day, but for those "survivors" who line these hallways.

If you think your day is going badly, simply spend some time in a nursing home.

I want us to visit these people, to give them hugs, to love them. Bring your kids, hold their hand. Just hold their hand. We have become such a disinfectant gel, hand-sanitizer society that we have forgotten the very basic tenet of love.

Touch.

Hold someone's hand, look into their eyes, and listen to their story. If there is no story, just hold their hand.

When I sit on the couch with my sons watching football, I often reach over and just hold their hands for no reason. This simple gesture shoots immediate warmth to my heart and tells my mind, their minds, "I love you" with nothing said. It offers an instant emotional connection and, oh, how it makes your heart feel.

Invariably, one of my sons will sink his head into the crook of my neck—no words exchanged, no deep glances, just this singular action. I feel so unbelievably content in these simple moments of love in my life that I want to bottle them because I know they will soon end with my boys ages fifteen, twelve, and ten. How much longer can they last?

Try this experiment with someone you love. It is so basic. Touch them, hold their hand, and follow the visceral feelings that shoot through your hand, up your arm, across your back, to your brain and heart; feel your body relax with warmth. If you stop and really follow this power through your body, you will see the raw power of simple touch and how it electrifies your body and soul. It is an unbelievable power.

Now, if it feels that powerful to you, imagine how it makes the other person feel. Human touch is the greatest life force in our world.

THE QUINTESSENCE OF LOVE

I think we all try to think of what we can "do" with the elderly— where we can take them, what activity they would like, what they might like to see—and that's all well and good.

But maybe we all overthink this. I say this from experience.

My grandfather and I would just hang out. We would maybe go to Friendly's and have an ice cream or a hamburger. We would talk about the Yankees and Mets; we would watch a ballgame and fall asleep on the couch together. We would just share each other's space. We laughed, we held hands when we walked, we always kissed goodbye. He was my greatest friend in life, and, in

LIFE IN 20 LESSONS

the smallness of those moments, he taught me so much more about the enduring power of love of a grandfather and grandson than I could only wish for others.

Some of my greatest memories of childhood were the days all three of us boys would visit my grandparents in Yonkers, New York, when my parents needed a break. I loved it. I got to sleep on the pullout couch with my brother. I could stay up a little later than usual. My Oma always made us an amazing meal, and she would have the best chocolates and Pepperidge Farm cookies stocked in the cupboard.

But on Saturdays, it was Opa's time with us. And it was generally the same thing. He would take us to Tibbetts Brook Park, and we would go for a walk. He would never drive into the park and pay admission. We would always find a side street and would cross a fence to enter the park (and my wife wonders where I get it from; so here, honey, here is where my frugality comes from). Then we would walk the park throwing a baseball or football and just talk.

Our favorite part of the walk was the brook that ran through the park. All three of us would craft a boat out of a stick we found on the ground, throw them in the brook, and watch as the current pushed our makeshift watercraft downstream. Then, the trash talking would begin as we taunted each other who would win this neophyte regatta. We each had long sticks we would use to navigate tough turns or larger water hazards like a clump of leaves or rocks. It was a race to the finish and super competitive with bragging rights for the weekend at stake.

I can remember like it was yesterday, looking over at my grandfather and seeing him smile as his three grandsons played next to him. He was in his element. To see him smiling back at me made me feel so loved. I could see it in his eyes. I could see the joy. Reflecting on it now, I know my Opa saw his brothers in us. I could see him remembering doing the same things with his brothers back in Germany all those years ago.

Perhaps the brook was a sad reminder of the angelic German village where he grew up. The family lived in the sawmill by a brook where two of his brothers tragically drowned. The town of Schlechtbach literally means "bad brook."

I know how much he loved his brothers and how his move to America was brutal on him. I know how much he enjoyed going back each year and then, as he got older, every few years. And then soon, he couldn't travel anymore. I thought of how sad he must have been being so far away from his brothers and sisters. One by one, we'd get the phone calls from Germany as they started to die.

As I sit here today and think about it, I wonder to myself, why did he never go back there? Why didn't he go and spend his waning years with his brothers and sisters all living together in their twilight? Why did he not do what would have been comfortable for him?

Because of us. Because of me, my brothers, and our mother. You talk about a love story.

My mother was an only child and, oh, what an amazing child she was to her father. My Oma died some years before Opa. The man was sixty-eight, and he would go on to live another twenty-two years without the woman he loved.

For what? For his daughter and his three grandsons.

Those days at Tibbetts Brook Park, I remember how happy my Opa was. I think of those days and how simple life was—a walk in the park with his grandsons. It didn't cost a dime and think of what I got. I got the memories in my head and the recollection of the times with my brothers and grandfather and how unbelievably amazing those days were.

May I just have one of those days back? Please, Lord, just give me one of those days as a small child with my brothers and my Opa walking in Tibbetts Brook Park. I want to see it once again. I want us to be all together just once more. I want for all of us to be locked in that moment, that space in time, that moment where my Opa looked deep into my eyes and said nothing, but really said everything I needed to know.

It takes no money, people. It takes no money at all. Children, grandchildren, they don't really want Disneyland. They don't want another Christmas gift under the tree. They want you. They want you, on the ground, at their eye level, doing the simple things you all love to do.

They just want you.

I can't be any more honest. I have experienced it as a child, and I have seen its reaction with my own children. Look into their eyes and they will see the love, share the words, embrace, hold them like you will never let go. The neurotransmitters in your brain will go into hyperdrive and you will feel an otherworldly connection.

The interpersonal stuff is the good stuff in this world. It is so simple. Listen to me, please, I beg of you, listen. I know the meaning of life and it is right here for all of us, for any of us to grasp. We are fooling ourselves to think it is anything different.

Your children are small only once. How many times has an older person said to you, "Enjoy it while it lasts"?

Because they know. They are living proof. As if they are real-life apparitions walking the streets to remind us what's good in life, what it all means.

It is right there in front of us. Stop. Get off the treadmill of life. Stop. Be with your family.

Our families are wherein our memories, past, present, and future, reside.

THE FIRST HORSEMAN CALLETH

A few years after his wife died, Opa moved up from Yonkers to Pleasantville to be closer to us. He bought a one-bedroom apartment less than a mile from our home and would come over for dinner a couple nights a week. He knew he needed to keep busy, so he became a driver at my dad's company, delivering engineering plans all over Westchester County. As the years went on, the distances got shorter and shorter, he slowly began turning down more and more requests for deliveries, and soon he retired—again.

A few years after that, he stopped driving at night, and soon thereafter started getting in progressively larger and larger accidents: first a fender bump, then a panel scratch, and finally some much closer and more serious calls. He was getting older and his reflexes were slowing down. My mom, dad, and I witnessed it most closely because we were there. But the realization came to my grandfather on his own. It was time to hang up his keys, at eighty-seven years of age.

We all assured him it would be no problem, but my parents had moved ten minutes farther away by then and the distance was noticeable. Why share this? Why tell you the story of my grandfather and his keys?

Because I want you all to understand this will be every one of us when the sun starts to set on our own lives. I often think of what must have been going through my grandfather's mind as he gave up those keys. I know the fear that must have been in his head. I know he must have felt he would be even more isolated.

Hanging up the keys is the one of most significant milestones of aging—the first horseman of the apocalypse.

Your world becomes markedly more local, limited by the distances you can now walk. You become more dependent on others to get to the store to buy groceries, run errands, and see friends. Hanging up the keys acts as the proverbial bucket of ice water to the face of your entire family. It puts everyone on notice that Grandpa is getting older; he will now need more help; and we will need to rally together. And, as the devoted child of a parent who gives up their keys, it is never enough. Psychologically, it is never enough, no matter how much you do. Your thoughts will always fill with "he is just sitting there alone, or I haven't heard from him today, does he have enough food."

In my family's particular circumstance, my mom couldn't sell her father's car for almost a year just out of respect and the possibility of a miracle that he would drive again. For my small part, I would pick him up and take him to my softball games to watch me play. We would grab some food together, and then I would bring him back home after a big night out.

In retrospect, I never did it enough. My guilt.

I distinctly remember the complete and utter joy on his face when he saw me pulling up. He would always already be standing outside, like an excited child waiting to go to his first ballgame. It's true, the circle of life. If I could just see that smile one more time, just once, as he entered my car and our eyes met before a quick hug and the smell of his Old Spice aftershave. (I am not embarrassed to tell you I need a bottle of Old Spice in my house at all times.)

I tell you this because the story is real. This whole story is real. I witnessed it all. I witnessed my grandfather's pain, his twilight, his slow descent into dementia, all the way until his last few hours.

I was there.

I want you all to know this story, not because I want you to know my grandfather, but because I want you to have empathy. Not for me, not for him, but for you. I want you to feel what he must have felt. I want you to understand, God willing, that will be you one day and that will be me.

What will you do? Who will you turn to?

My wish is we start today. Empathize with the millions of elderlies exactly in my grandfather's shoes, living today. If not your own family, there are millions of others who need you. There are so many. And we can help them. You can help them. You don't even need a reason.

I encourage all families to foster relationships with the grand-parents, aunts, uncles, and the elderly in your community. It teaches our children so many virtues, but the greatest gifts it teaches are reverence, dignity, compassion, and empathy.

We all get old...eventually. And getting old is not always pretty. Getting older with the spark and vitality of children and family surrounding you? That is far, far better.

IN SUM

We need to reconnect with the elderly of this country. We need to visit, to engage, to hold their hands. We will bring joy to their days, and, in doing so, we will have empathy for them; we will see ourselves in their shoes; our children will see us in their shoes. We will all be there one day, God willing. And we can't wait. We need to do it now, before it's too late.

We can do this. We are equipped. At least we can try. It won't be easy. Those things that aren't easy usually hold the greatest reward. The elderly of this country need us to reconnect with them. To remember them. To be cared about, to simply be touched. Let's all take this upon our collective selves. I have seen it firsthand. We are too strong a nation, too strong a people, too wealthy a country to treat our elderly like this. Visit, touch, engage, listen. It will be all of us one day.

THE REMINDERS

The elderly need us.

––––––––––

Taking care of each other is the circle of life.

––––––––––

Your children will benefit.

––––––––––

Empathy, above all, have empathy.

––––––––––

We will all be them one day.

––––––––––

18 Exercise Your Mind

My parents are eighty. They did it. They retired early, lived by the beach, and traveled the globe more than I could ever dream of. They are rock stars. Not only did they give me the greatest childhood a boy could ever ask for, they made a difference in so many people's lives, and they retired exactly as they wanted to. For two children of immigrants from the South Bronx, they frickin' crushed it! And, thank you, Lord, they are still healthy.

And we talk. We talk about things in their now eightieth year. We mostly talk about...

PLAYING DEFENSE
And just how I preach to my boys when playing basketball, defense wins championships.

You're lucky to make it to eighty years of age. Depending on who you believe, you are lucky. Supreme athletes die randomly in their twenties. Yet my grandmother lived on butter and whipped cream and lived till ninety-nine. A child is stricken with cancer and dies at six. A neighbor drinks gin from morning till night and lives past 100. No one really knows.

Now, you're still healthy, but you see yourself slowing down. There are more aches and pains. You're sleeping more. The same energy of just a few years ago just isn't there. Driving long distances doesn't hold the same allure. Jet lag seems harsher and more tedious. Meals on your trips start to affect your belly. And you are attending more funerals in your social set.

As you lie in bed after a particularly long day, you start to do the simple math of our grade school years in your head.

How many good years do I have left? What constitutes a good year?

Who will take care of me? I don't want to be a burden to my kids.

You figure eighty to eighty-five years of age might be reasonable to expect; anything after eighty-five is gravy.

This starts the "playing defense" years.

But I say fight it! Fight it every step of the way.

My retiree brothers and sisters, here it is in three simple steps:

1. You must exercise your mind daily with positive stimuli: music, film, art, reading, crossword puzzles, sudoku, anything that challenges your mind. Do not plop down on your La-Z-Boy and watch TV. That is tantamount to placing one foot in the grave. If your day becomes routine, your life will be shorter. Mix it up and move. Stop simply saying, "I am getting older, I forgot." Remember! Challenge yourself to remember dates,

names, grocery lists, and directions. It might feel ridiculous, but it is a worthwhile exercise. An idle mind is not only the devil's workshop, it is death's companion.

2. Interact with humans. Converse, go to lunch, movies, church, knitting group, book club, socialize, socialize, socialize. I don't have the heart to tell you the stories of those "clients" who have worked their whole lives only to retire and die six months later. Get out among people and talk!

3. Lastly (and I truly believe this because I see it with my own parents), share your life experience with your community or someone just starting out. Mentor an aspiring businessperson in an organization like SCORE or your local Chamber of Commerce. Coach or tutor a family member, a friend's child, someone. Have them for dinner, work out a plan together, become vested in their cause. You will both benefit and make the world a better place in the process. This sharing of knowledge makes us all stronger, better, more powerful. And when it's not done via a computer, communication becomes more personal, more human. Better.

There is greatness in these encounters, and you will exercise your mind in the process.

THE ALBATROSS MUST DIE

And to my younger brothers and sisters—

It's done. Over. No more.

Society has told us to play it out like this: After high school, we must go to college, after college, grad, business, law, med, whatever school.

I think we may want to rethink this as a society.

I realize it is easy for me to say already having my degrees. I get it. And, yes, my higher education has given me the confidence, and the street cred, to say, "I am an attorney," undeniably. I have had the privilege (yes, it is a privilege) to have had my parents and grandparents pay for all of my education. A privilege not everyone has, and there are way smarter people out there who deserve to be able to go to school, if they wish. Way smarter!

In many cases, I simply do not believe the diploma is worth the cost of the paper it is written on. Yet society, and employers, still judge us based on that diploma. Therein lies the grand dilemma.

My main problem with higher education is the albatross of personal debt it causes. Unless, and until, we figure out a higher education system that does not burden our youth and its families as it currently does, I favor work experience over higher education in all instances.

I would encourage all kids to find a thriving company in a field/discipline you are curious about, get in on the ground floor (just get in), and do not worry about the salary because you are, most likely, not worth anything to the company.

Starting out, you will be taking up a chair, a desk, a stapler, and oxygen. Just being real, I was there.

Then, show up fifteen minutes early every single day, turn off your cell phone and place it aside until lunchtime, look people in the eye when you speak with them, provide them with a firm

handshake, be competent and accountable to your superiors, educate yourself while there in any way possible (companies will pay
to make you smarter; it benefits them), somehow prove your worth
to the company (otherwise, why be there?), learn to listen (Let me
say this again, **learn to listen**; it is the greatest gift in the world.),
go above and beyond in all that you do, and be kind. Kindness
above all!

Never, I mean never, just collect a paycheck; it hurts you in the
long run.

Pretty simple, right?

And here's the kicker. If you truly are any good, companies will
see that, and some will pay for your education; just ask my wife.

Parents, if you have the means to send your child to college,
make certain they are ready to go. We are all so different, so unique.
Do not send your seventeen- or eighteen-year-old to college if they
are not ready for it. Let your child work, figure it out, and see how
hard the world is. And make them pay rent if they live at home (my
parents made me). I guarantee that child will grow up fast and beg
you to go to college to learn. The most difficult part will be looking
inward at yourself as a parent to see if you are confident enough
to tell your neighbors, or friends at a cocktail party, your child is
"figuring it out." You'll soon find out, it is not just a kid issue.

I saw it firsthand with my brother who wasn't ready to go off
to college. He pulled a Blutarsky and got a 0.00—not easy to do.

He is now a doctor.

Do not underestimate street smarts, will, and life experience.

CREATE

And for all ages—

I believe what makes America great is we are among the best inventors in the world. We are a creation nation.

Yes, I am biased, but I believe there is something in the air here that makes people feel as if anything is possible. I am uncertain what it is. Seeing so many people succeed from nothing, hearing the manifold immigrant stories upon which our country was founded, the rags-to-riches mentality of the nation? It's in the soil. This creation can be in business or art or music or processes. It doesn't matter the field because creating something gives you a huge sense of accomplishment, no matter how small or seemingly insignificant.

SIDEBAR WARNING! If you decide to create something with another human being, family or otherwise, you must have legal documents drawn up PRIOR to starting anything that indicates a clear delineation of ownership and, preferably, all parties' time commitment to the cause, which is always difficult to quantify. Without that, I would not advise putting in one hour of work toward your common goal. I am sorry, there are simply no exceptions to this rule (watch *The Social Network*, Columbia Pictures, 2010, for a case in point).

I can say this with all candor and experience because I created something from absolutely nothing but an idea in my head, while sitting in the backroom of a funeral home in a small town in California.

I owned three funeral homes over a ten-year period. I would see a market and go after it, buy some real estate, set up a funeral home. In those ten years, I applied for and received fourteen loans of all types: commercial and residential real estate, equipment, lines of credit, auto loans. You name it, I got it. Each time I would go through the same process to obtain a loan: collect three years of my personal and corporate tax returns of every entity in which I had at least 33 percent ownership, prepare personal financial statements (basically a detailed list of every asset and every liability I owned and owed), gather all "official" corporate documents (incorporation papers, articles, statements of information, state and local business licenses, and so on), and fill out a bank's lengthy and detailed application.

In my case, the volume of paper I was required to give to just one bank looked like three Tolstoy novels stacked on top of each other. I would then make copies of all of these most private documents only to hand them over to a twenty-seven-year-old banker who would, in turn, give them to his bank's underwriter. Nine times out of ten, I would never see these documents again—my most private information. Gone!

In order to obtain the best rate for my loans, I would do this process with three to five banks for each loan I needed, and I would await their offers (known as "term sheets"), which set out the particulars of the loan the bank would be willing to give me. It was a necessary exercise that took an inordinate amount of time away from running my businesses, and I felt the banks knew most people would not want to take as much time to find the best rate for their loan.

I thought the loan process was flawed and unfairly skewed against me, and I didn't like that. I didn't think that was fair. I felt that banks had the upper hand in this negotiation (the most important investment of most of our lives), and I wanted to level the playing field for everybody.

I thought I could create something to make it easier, faster, certainly more fair (ya know, because I had all this banking, coding, and financial expertise already... not!). So I mocked up a prototype and hired a friend to create a website for me. I showed it to a buddy, whom I thought could bring some technical expertise. He said my site sucked (an accurate, if offensive statement), but, together, we could build something way better.

And we did.

Over four years later, we have www.magillaloans.com, an anonymous loan search engine that better educates borrowers about the largest investment of their lives—whether their home or business. I was an unemployed screenwriter turned funeral home owner who had the idea to create a fintech (financial technology) platform to change the way we do loans in the world.

Be that crazy!

Get up off your ass and create. You have it in you. I am telling you it exists inside there; that brilliant idea is just currently lying dormant.

If I can do it, anything is possible. We are, after all, a creation nation.

WILL IT

Sometimes, to create, we need inspiration. I like books on the power of positive thinking. I believe it works. You place thoughts in your mind, envision your plan, couple that with action, and will it to happen. It sounds insane, but the process works—for me.

Here was my go-to list of books:

- Norman Vincent Peale's *The Power of Positive Thinking*
- Rhonda Byrne's *The Secret*
- Napoleon Hill's *Think and Grow Rich*
- *The Greatest Salesman in the World* by Og Mandino
- Stephen R. Covey's *The Seven Habits of Highly Effective People*
- Dale Carnegie's *How to Win Friends and Influence People*
- Zig Ziglar on *Secrets of Closing the Sale*

I have taken principles from each of these authors and implemented them into my life. In sum, an exercise of my mind: think it, visualize it (getting a little New Age-y here), put it out into the universe, and finally act—you *must* add action.

I am not talking about just sitting in the corner and trying to use The Force; that's not realistic. But you can "will" things to happen.

I wanted to transfer back East and go to college near my brother. Done.

I wanted to go to law school. Done.

I wanted to make a movie. Done.

I wanted to be a screenwriter in LA. Done.

I wanted to marry a great woman. Done.

I wanted to be a great dad. Still trying.

I wanted to create an internet site. Done.

I wanted to write a book. Done, done, and frickin' done!

I "willed" those things to happen, and I ain't even that bright. Success won't just happen on its own. But if you have no connections and just sheer will, your mind mixed with action will make it happen. You just push all negative thoughts out of your head; you train your mind to never hear no; you never listen to a parent's friend or family member laugh when you suggest what you want to do at Thanksgiving dinner. You put all the doubters and naysayers out of your mind and forge onward.

Or better yet, look those doubters right in the eye and just stare for a beat. In that moment, remember their face so, when you succeed, you can remember it with a smile.

I've got a yearbook full of doubters in my mind.

Look, I am not book smart. I can't read something once and know it. I never took standardized tests well nor do I know the particular inner workings of the human mind, but I can tell you this from my own experience, you can "will" what you want to happen.

If you believe it, it can happen. What do you want to make happen?

———

IN SUM

Whether we are young or old, we need to exercise our minds. Our brain is like a muscle and muscles need to be worked. This becomes more apparent as we age simply because our minds are, generally, not used as much; our body functions slow down; and there is more idle time to fill our days.

If you are older, surround yourself with activity and youth; if you are younger, surround yourself with experience and knowledge. These types of relationships can only foster greatness. The higher education of our youth is on its way out in favor of more pragmatic experience, creating, and inventing. America is very good at inventing.

We made the Pringle, right?

And we are lucky because it is easier than ever to educate ourselves. Khan Academy (www.khanacademy.org), Master-Class, and their various offshoots, give us all the ability to learn more and learn anew. There should, never again, be a question of inability to educate ourselves, if the willingness is there; it is now a mouse click away. (Now let's get everyone the ability to have that mouse click.) Similarly, YouTube videos can teach us almost anything under the sun. Explore audiobooks, podcasts, TED Talks, blogs, webinars, NPR, vlogs, MOOCs, continuing ed classes at community colleges, college classes to audit, Osher Lifelong Learning Institute—there are no longer impediments to keeping our minds sharp.

Exercise your mind!

THE REMINDERS

It is easier than ever to exercise our minds.

If you are older, surround yourself with youth; if you are younger, surround yourself with experience.

Create! Whatever you love, create.

The power of positive thinking works.

Will things to happen.

---

19 Be Resilient

What if you were told your child will die in the next five to ten years?

What if you were told there is no cure?

What if you were told they would be uncomfortable as their disease progressed?

What would you do?

We had bonded with the family from afar. Both of our sons had hearing impairments. When this new family came to our school, the administration called us to see if we would share our story with them. Our son used an FM system in the classroom to help him hear the teacher more clearly, and they wanted to pick our brains.

That is all we were told.

Angie met the mom and downloaded all she knew. The family was grateful, and they shared all the ideas and treatments they were doing to help their son.

This family was dialed in. The dad was a doctor, and the mom was one of those people who just had it all locked down. She was no joke. She knew everything about anything related to her son's hearing loss and the ramifications of all its potential surrounding areas.

There was no stone unturned; in fact, my wife came home and started questioning if we were doing enough. This woman had that much breadth of knowledge.

We never became close friends because our children were in different classes and sometimes that's just how it works out. But we always felt a kindred spirit toward their family.

A few years later they left our school. I thought that was odd because our school was a tightly knit bunch of families where a child who was a little different could always fit in. We heard their son needed more care, something the other school was better equipped for. Years later we heard their son had a rare auditory condition (dystopia deafness syndrome) that only seven documented children had worldwide—and there was no known cure.

This hit home to us. This was a family we thought was more like us than most because we shared the commonality of our sons' hearing loss and now we were being told their child would die in a matter of years.

What do you do as a parent? How do you live each day knowing that your child's timeline is ticking before your eyes?

And to further complicate matters, your child is in pain on a daily basis. You want to be with them and live each day, to love them every minute you can.

The best of the best children's hospitals have tried all their last resorts. You have exhausted every means possible. But you continue to search and pray—pray that someone, somewhere, will come out of the medical shadows and say, "I found it!"

You pray that day will come. But it doesn't.

And your child is in pain. Excruciating pain. And you see it, every day. Do you pray for your child to be taken from this pain when there is no cure? When you want their pain to stop? When the doctors have told you they have exhausted every possible operation, idea, technique?

Easy if it's not your child. Be human, please, Lord, take the child out of their pain. But this is YOUR child. YOUR everything. How can the world make anyone's mind have to go through this and then still try to do all the regular life stuff like hold a job, take care of other kids, yourself, go to the grocery store, shower.

Every single detail is profoundly impacted.

How cruel. How unfair. How heartless.

We have friends who are way closer to this family than we are. They have shared the family's struggles. But, really, how can any of us know what truly goes on when the friends step out the front door and it's just the family to live the other twenty-two hours of the day? The other 166 hours of the week? The other 670 hours of the month, the year?

There is only resilience.

GET UP!

Back in the day, there was a boxer named Gerry Cooney. He was a big Irish Catholic guy, about 6 feet 7, known for his powerful punches and a 28–3 career record, losing two of those three in heavyweight title bouts in the early 1980s.

When he fought, it always seemed like a war, and he would be a bloody mess, sometimes even getting knocked down. He fought guys like Norton, Holmes, Spinks, and Foreman—some say the golden age of boxers. I only know this because my grandfather loved boxing. I have no idea why such a peaceful man loved to watch two men beat each other senseless, but he loved it.

Anyway, my Opa really admired Gerry Cooney, and I could never understand it. As I remember it, Cooney never truly got the recognition he may have deserved, in the Larry Holmes era. While he may have never been the greatest fighter in history, he earned my Opa's respect, and I'm certain that of millions more boxing fans because he just kept coming no matter how many times he got knocked down.

And if this story of resilience can be used as a grander metaphor for our lives, it would be perfect.

We get beaten down by people, by circumstances, by life. It happens. It will happen. It happens to everyone at some point(s) in each of our lives. But if we just keep getting up, even if we don't win, think of what that says to the world? I threw my hardest stuff at this guy and he keeps coming back for more.

Things happen on all of our journeys. There is sickness and death, abuse and addiction, betrayal and infidelity, heartbreak and anguish, bad stuff in everyone's lives, over a lifetime. But from these challenging times comes overcoming adversity, obstacles, and growth, and those experiences breed physical and mental toughness. That is the good stuff that makes life worth living.

"It is not how many times you are knocked down; it is how many times you get up" was attributed to either Colonel George Custer or former Green Bay Packer Coach Vince Lombardi. These wise words could be the greatest quote in the history of mankind.

To me, it has nothing to do with sports but, rather, defines the human condition, the story of life. Look no further than *Rocky*, *Rudy*, or *Shawshank Redemption*—movies about the the enduring human spirit. It is why we are human; we endure against all odds.

You have heard the stories of many people who failed multiple times before they became successful. Look it up and see manifold failures in the lives of Henry Ford, Thomas Edison, Abe Lincoln, Van Gogh, Dr. Seuss, Ben Franklin—the list from history is endless.

And you are in your history right now, as we speak. No one knocks it out of the park the first time, no matter what you've heard. Their successes, whatever they were, were because of resiliency.

IF I AM BEING HONEST

I am writing a book about life's meaning and how I learned all of these valuable lessons along my journey, but I need to be crystal clear: I am far from this scholarly being that walks this earth with Gandhi-like serenity.

The reality is I suffer from anxiety.

I have the exact life I want, yet I suffer from anxiety. I have not been clinically diagnosed, but I know I suffer. There is sleeplessness and worry. There are times when I awaken with seeming heart palpitations and neck sweating. I swear I feel stiffness in my arms, ya know the onset of a stroke or a grand mal. Upon reflection they are in times of stress about business, doing too much, and just general worrying.

And these anxieties are very real.

I went on my son's field trip to the art museum. I talked to another dad. He told me he suffers from anxiety and depression.

He uses meds. He seemingly has a great life: multiple shops all running well, nice home, nice car, happy wife, great kids.

"What the hell are you anxious about?" I asked him.

"You know, what this all means, how I am gonna pay for college. Life."

"But you do yoga. No, you *teach* yoga. You are my ultimate zen master."

"Nah, dude, the yoga gets me more in tune, focuses me, and then I get even more anxious and depressed about things."

I burst out laughing.

"Your father helped you out with all this, right? Taught you how to cope?" He sarcastically chimed in already knowing the answer.

I laughed even harder.

"So, what's the answer? What do you really want to do?" I asked.

He looked deeply into my eyes and was as serious as the heart attack I always think I'm having: "Ski."

"What?"

"Ski. Work for the mountain, make a hundred and twenty, pay cash for everything."

And if this weren't at least the third conversation I have had with a dad in the last year, I wouldn't think anything of it. Is this a way more pervasive problem then we all realize?

So I got to thinking about what middle-aged men are anxious about and why this anxiety is as widespread as I know it is. As an exercise, I sat down and enumerated my anxieties in hopes that this would, in some way, purge the feeling from inside of me—you know, mature stuff, like if I talk about my fears, it would be healthy, good for me, that whole cathartic thing.

Yeah, it didn't. But maybe it is helpful to understand a growing epidemic in America, if not the world.

So what am I anxious about?

My children—

How will they grow up?

Am I doing enough to shape them?

Am I giving them enough independence?

Will they fall in love?

Do they rely on my wife and me too much?

Are they spoiled?

Can they hold a conversation with an adult?

Will I be able to pay for their college?

Is college even right for each of them?

Will health be an issue?

Am I strict enough?

Am I too strict?

Are they lazy?

Are their grades good enough?

Am I doing enough?

My family—

Are my parents okay?

Are they happy?

I should talk to my siblings more.

What should we do when family come visit?

Do I see everyone enough?

How much longer will my parents be on this earth?

What happens if one of them dies first?

Would they move in with me?

I should talk to my brother about our problems.

I couldn't have them in an assisted-living facility.

I want them near me.

My job—

Do I want to do this the rest of my life?

What else would I do?

Could I make enough to support our family if I did that?

Could I move the family just for my new job?

Would they all be happy?

Do I have enough savings?

Do I have enough for college tuition?

Do I have enough for retirement?

My wife—

Is she happy?

Am I doing enough for her?

Do we have enough alone time?

Does she have enough time away from me?

Does she need that purse?

How can I be a better husband?

Does she know how much I love her?

Why shouldn't she have that purse?

Me—

Am I truly happy?

Am I a good son, father, husband, brother, human?

What does this life all mean?

Do I exercise enough?

Why didn't the Vikings draft a left tackle?

Do I have enough me time?

I shouldn't eat that cake.

Does my wife still find me attractive?

Why shouldn't I eat that cake?

I don't want to bore you all by reading my full list, so I simply scratched the surface. I realize some of you are saying, "Slowly back away from the keyboard and dial 911," while others are saying "middle-class problems." I should shut my mouth, I have food, safety, and shelter.

Word.

My point? We all got problems, just different ones. No one gets off easy.

IN SUM

It is unfortunate, but you will have difficult times in your life. It is unfortunate, but it will be your reality; no one gets a smooth sailing pass through life. It simply does not exist. But when you are down, if you simply dig deep, roll over, and get back up, think of what that says to the world. You have seen this a thousand times before from heroes, antiheroes, monsters, armies, whomever, in movies, literature, and life.

It's the fight, the resiliency, the enduring human spirit that exists inside us all. It's in there waiting to be called into action. The question is, are you able to say yes to this new beginning?

And I bet if you asked a thousand successful people—business leaders, preachers, teachers, nurses, social workers, whomever—every single one of them will tell you the struggle, the climb, the getting there, that is the good the stuff. The times when you had to grind all day not knowing the outcome, obstacle after obstacle in your way, uncertain if you will succeed or fail. Because, in the end, that is what we remember.

The "how we got here," the dash (the life you live between your birth date and your expiration date), that is the real story, the story people want to hear about, marvel at, respect, and maybe that is where you currently are in life—trying to figure out how to succeed.

And now it's time to finish your story, to push through what's blocking you (we all have something) and finish your story.

What are you waiting for?

THE REMINDERS

*It is not how many times you get knocked down,
it is how many times you get back up.*

Someone has it worse than you—guaranteed.

---

*When you are face down in the gutter, simply
roll over and all you see is stars.*

---

*National Suicide Prevention Lifeline, call
(800) 273-8255, available 24/7.*

20 DEST (Do Epic Shit Today)

You are going to die. Read that again. You *are* going to die.

I pray it is peacefully in your sleep when you are ninety-seven and up to that very evening you were of sound mind and your body was fully functional and you just finished an amazing dinner with your entire family and closest friends, and everyone hugged and kissed you and told you of the depths of their enduring love for you.

But you ain't goin' out like that.

Our lots in life are probably going to be much different. I am sorry to be the bearer of this bad news, but I have lived it for the last fourteen years, and I have not been to one home, or met with one family, in which that scenario has happened.

More likely are the events surrounding death that make life so cruel and unfair: a protracted illness plays out with a slow descent to the end; a healthy man has a heart attack on his bike ride; a child is stricken with leukemia; a mother dies before her children reach middle school; a father suffers a fatal stroke while on vacation with his children; a son drowns while abalone fishing; a daughter is killed instantly in an auto wreck with her girlfriends—a simple slip and fall, gunshots, the list is as endless as it is tragic.

Sobering, right?

I think the major common theme from surviving members of families I have heard is this: Live your life the way you wish to live it. That way, when it is all said and done, you and your surviving loved ones will have no regrets. You will end it all with a smile on your face and a life well lived.

In my life experience in the death industry, the families who feel less sadness and pain are those who know their loved one did exactly that. They lived the life they wanted to live with no excuses and no regrets. Conversely, the most regret I saw from families was when they wanted something more for that person; they wished they had helped them live a better life; they wished they put the pettiness aside and made amends before it was too late.

This is the best advice I can give you knowing what I know. Live your life the exact way you want to live it. If you think it can't be done, you are simply wrong. I have seen too many fantastic miracles in this world to believe otherwise. Your mind will take you there. I know this for certain.

Heed the stories before us, the others who have made mistakes, of those who have regrets. They are our greatest teachers. Go and live the life you want. Now!

Go! Now!

THE STATUS QUO IS DEAD

Our world is filled with conventional thinkers. In fact, there is a conventional way society tells us to go through life: go to college, get a job, marry, have 2.3 kids, buy a house with a picket fence, take two weeks of vacation a year, retire, collect social security, and die.

You know what? I ain't going out like that—and neither should you.

I want you to forget the status quo, what you think society expects of you, and what your parents, or others, want you to do.

Convention blows.

I want you to think differently and create. Remember, failure is good. Think of these dudes: da Vinci, Edison, the Wright brothers, Wozniack, Brinn, Page, Musk, and Bezos. You think those dorks sat around lamenting going to college and finding the right mate? You think they didn't fail a hundred times (or more) before knocking that shit out of the park? You think they sat around their crappy apartment eating Cheetos in their underpants? Well...

No!

I know their minds, and this is how they think: failure, tweak, failure, tweak, failure, tweak, failure, tweak, until no more failure, until it fails again; then tweak, failure, tweak, failure, tweak...

Look, I just created your own personal roadmap. Go live it, and stop being such a puss.

SO HOW DO I START?

First, stop whining.

Next, ask yourself two questions: What if...? and Why not me?

"What if...I created a better mousetrap?"

"What if...there were a better breakfast cereal than the one I am currently eating?"

"What if...humans could breathe on Mars?"

"What if... [insert any idea/curiosity/dream you feel passionate about in your own life]?"

Do you see where I am headed with this?

If you constantly ask yourself the simple question of "What if?" the seeds of a great idea are germinated. The "What if" question is the genesis of all great inventions in this world and is the spark of all initial creativity in every human.

Now, the "What if" question should always be immediately followed by a second question: "Why not me?"

"Why would I leave this for someone else to discover or create?"

"Why not me?"

I believe most of the world comes to a collective halt before this question; I think most people give up here and just stop. But what if we all asked, "Why not me?" Think of the possibilities we could create.

But, Chris, I am living in a shit-box apartment on the outskirts of Topeka, how could I—

STOP!

Why NOT you?

Stop listening to the media, to Mom and Dad, or worry what

people might think you should do. You are the only you, you dictate where your car is going. If someone doesn't believe in you, prove them wrong. If you don't get into the best school, prove to them that someone from any school, or no school, can succeed.

And why would school even matter with all that is available to us on the internet, in libraries, or in our mentors' minds? You are the master of your own journey. Do not let anyone else drive your car. Get in the driver's seat, strap in, and drop the frickin' hammer!

Why NOT you?

PARENTS OF THE WORLD

You can help. You can really help with all this.

Look, we're all scared. Honestly, we are all scared our children will be losers, marry the wrong person, or live in our basement forever, and never provide us with any grandchildren.

I get it. I have all of those same fears…and more.

Have you ever heard your child say this? "But I don't know what I want to do with my life." Only every single parent across the entire globe forever in time, right? So here's where it gets good. Next time you hear that from a child, get up in their grill, look them right in the eye, and shout, "DEST!"

Huh?

"DEST! Do Epic Shit Today!"

It means aspire to greatness. It means think above your pay grade. It means constantly ask yourself "What if?" and "Why not me?" If we start out thinking like this, I guarantee good things are going to happen over our lifetimes.

DEST, baby!

IN SUM

These times we are currently living in are the most epic ever. With the internet, our world has become smaller and smaller and given us more, and quicker, access to everything faster than ever before. The educational opportunities available to us all at the click of a mouse are so fantastic the mind cannot even conceive of how easy it is to learn. But that is only half the battle. The rest must come from within. The "What if" takes research, the "Why not me?" takes action. Learn, act, make mistakes, tweak, and never fear what lies ahead because it all works out.

Trust me, in the end, it all works out.

THE REMINDERS

"What if" you did something you loved your whole life?

Why someone else? Why not you?

Do Epic Shit...TODAY!

When it's all said and done, let's close our eyes
for the last time with a smile on our faces.

THE LESSONS

Be Thankful

Make a Difference

Avoid Judgment

Respect Others and Yourself

Be Vulnerable

Get Uncomfortable

Failure Is the Foundation

Love Simply

Become a Famillionaire

Make a Few Good Friends

Be with Self

Laugh

Enjoy Food

Sweat, Fiber, and Water

Stop Worrying about Money

Have Faith or Spirituality

Embrace the Elderly

Exercise Your Mind

Be Resilient

DEST

The Big Finish

You, dear reader, may ask this: *So, what now, funeral man? We have come all this way with you. We have listened. We have closed our mouths and listened. Now tell us. Tell us about the inconsolable pain of losing someone you truly love. Give us the professional opinion, the sage advice from the funeral guy, the guy who has seen so much. What did you discover about life in the death industry?*

First, I hope you have felt that inconsolable pain because it means you have truly loved. Like a part of you is missing. Like a pit at the base of your stomach that disables your desire for food or sunlight or movement.

And it lasts. Oh, how it lasts.

That pain is commensurate with the amount you have loved—extreme pain, extreme love. Congratulations if you have felt that.

But let's be real.

I have read all of the books on grieving and loss: John Gunther's *Death Be Not Proud*, Elisabeth Kubler-Ross *On Death & Dying*, the poem "The Dash" by Linda Ellis, Rabbi Harold Kushner's *When Bad Things Happen to Good People*, *How We Die* by Sherwin B.

Nuland, *Being Mortal* by Atul Gawande, and, of course, I know well the famous expression "time heals all wounds."

Bullshit! Total and utter bullshit!

Sure the pain subsides over time because there comes a day when you look in the mirror at the shell of the person you have become, and you hear your loved one say—

Come on now. Stay strong. Pick yourself up. Enough. I am okay. You gotta keep living. You gotta move on with your life. I know you love me, and I love you too…endlessly. I know how much you miss me, and please know how much I miss you too. I will wait. I will wait here for you. I will wait here for you and when it is your time, we shall be together again. For all of eternity. We will meet again. We shall love again. I am not afraid. I am warm. I am comforted. I am…okay. And I am with you. I am here, but I am with you. You may not see me, you may not feel me, you may not touch me, but I am here. I am with you.

There comes that day. I promise. I promise that day comes. And when it does, you will know. You will know that you need to carry on. To move on.

But the real question people want to know after the death of a loved one is this: How do you cope?

My professional opinion after living it, seeing it, reading all the renowned authorities in the field is this: You don't.

Awesome. I paid twenty-five bucks, read this whole damn book, and then that.

See, you simply live with loss, it comes in waves, and you emotionally body surf those waves; sometimes you are at one with the
wave as it breaks at that perfect spot just behind the curl, and you
ride it seamlessly in and it gently glides you toward the shoreline
with ease among the white foam and bubbles of the now receding
water around you. At other times, you get caught ahead of the
curl, you feel the back of your feet rise, and the surge slams you
to the ocean floor almost shattering your neck as you tumble and
scrape the sand, ass over tea kettle, praying you make it back to the
surface so you can breathe again.

Time heals all wounds?

Sure, maybe the freshness of death subsides, and it stings a
little less as your sun rises increase. But, in my opinion, we are
changed forever. Forever changed. We are never the same person.
How could we be?

I have said many times, to anyone who will listen, the harshest
aspect about death is that life continues around you: There are still
people in line at Starbucks; traffic doesn't abate; people don't stay
in their houses and observe a few days of collective mourning for
your loved one.

Life keeps on going no different than the day before, except
your world has been forever altered in this morass of humans
around you.

That is not fair. That is what they call life. That is where you
have heard this phrase: Life is not fair.

It isn't, it truly isn't.

That is why you must grieve on your own schedule, and no two
schedules are the same. My grief cannot be compared to your grief

because I may have felt differently about my grandfather than you felt about yours. My experiences with him were unique to us and now he is gone.

In many ways grieving is similar to dieting. How the heck do I know how to lose weight with your body? You know better than anyone else, because your fat pants are now tight or the jeans you always wanted to get into now fit like a glove.

It's the same with grieving. Only you know your grief cycle based on your own intimate and unique experiences with the loved one who has died. There can be no other explanation.

There is no how-to manual. THIS is no how-to manual. I cannot know the pain that is unique to you.

Sure, the stages of grief are a nice generalization, but your stages may be different than the next person's or may be missing a few or have additional stages no book has mentioned because... they are your own!

Case in point, my grandfather. I don't know how my brothers felt when he died. Sure, they were sad, they grieved, they missed him, but I do not know the extent of their pain. I don't even want to guess.

I simply know my pain because I ate lunch with him regularly, I had dinner with him, and he came to my softball games with regularity. I probably saw him way more than they did. I enjoyed his company. I invited him over when my parents were away just to sit and watch football with me. We often did nothing together. We didn't have to. We loved one another, and we were friends.

I cried many nights after his death, and to this day, some twenty years later, I tear up when I think of him. And I think of him often.

And let me tell you how it goes down.

My grandfather loved the outdoors. He was raised in a sawmill and had to travel by horse and carriage into the woods to drag trees out of the forest to be cut and sold. It was crazy hard work and long, hard days. I can't even imagine. But you know what he remembered in each of those days? How beautiful and peaceful the forest was.

The guy was dragging timber out of the forest with nothing more than a horse, carriage, and some ropes, and he was finding beauty in the trees.

My grandfather took each one of his grandsons to Germany alone, as a treat. He showed us where he grew up. We stayed with his sisters across from the former sawmill the family operated. He walked each of us, individually, into the forest where he got those trees. To this day, I remember our walk out there. I remember his face as he looked around the trees, clearly remembering those "woebegone" days with his brothers, in this very same forest, with reverence and love.

When I was there, he was lost in thought. He teared up and then remembered I, his fourteen-year-old grandson, was staring up at him. He put his arm around me and said, "Ya, Christ, those were the days." (He called me "Chris" in his broken English, and it came out as "Chris-t." How's that for pressure?)

People, I don't know. I don't know how you cope. I am not a learned man. I really am not. I will tell you this, though. I go for walks around my neighborhood in the early morning, before the world starts. It is quiet. It is real damn quiet, and no one is around. Trees are everywhere and I feel my grandfather way more than I want to admit. I hear him. I smell him. Jesus, sometimes I feel so close to him, I expect him to walk out of the trees as I pass by.

See, I don't cope. I feel him all around me to this very day. And when I get back home, I kneel next to my sons' beds, kiss their cheeks, and tell them it is time to get up for school.

I wish my boys knew my Opa. But I am grateful they know their Papa and Grampy.

Forget the coping. Tell people when they are here, today, in your presence, while you have the chance. Let loved ones know, today, how much they mean to you. It will ease your pain when they are gone. No regrets as you stand at their funeral service, and I've seen way too many of those regrets.

That much I can guarantee you.

I have talked about death a lot in this book. Forgive me, it was my profession for an amazingly wonderful part of my life. For me, it has been the catalyst to a deeper appreciation for life and my family. Family means everything to me, literally everything. But I am certain you have seen that if you are reading this.

I have really loved writing this book. Thank you for reading it.

For My Boys

My greatest joy, the only thing I have ever truly wanted to be, my true and complete happiness, is being your dad. Just know this forever and ever.

I fear nothing. I have you.

I am living the greatest life anyone could ever ask for being your dad. I have gotten to coach every single one of you, in all kinds of sports, been to every performance at school, made every open house, and loved every moment of it. I have won with you and we have lost together, some truly tremendous wins and some really crushing defeats. In many ways this is a microcosm of life, and now you are prepared. Life doesn't always go your way.

Love and family are the answer. With those two, all else falls in line.

Sure, you need to work, but I implore you to do something you love that fits your lifestyle; never forsake your family for a job; no money, no accolades, no possessions are worth that. Not in this lifetime, not in any lifetime. And that's hard to understand starting out because the media and society seem to tell us differently.

Don't listen.

DO. NOT. LISTEN!

I know by now you all know you are the greatest loves of my life. I know you do. I would give you my last breath to be with you forever. And we will be with each other forever and ever. I am certain of that. Supremely certain. You can take that to the bank.

When our time is done, I promise you there is a greater place, so great we cannot even fathom its greatness, in a far better place, and this place is already pretty awesome.

You come from great people. Your grandparents, on both sides, are tremendous human beings: generous, giving, kind, loving, and all about family. They too believe in a Higher Power. This will help you in life. You come from a solid foundation, and you will build on what they have already given us—memory brick by memory brick and a shit ton of love.

I want you all to never feel sorry for me in any way. I am living the exact life I want to live, and I am frickin' crushing it. What a great time I had, and am having, with you. And what amazing people I have met. But none greater than you and your mom. My complete joys, the incarnate of love.

I am so excited to grow old with you and cheer you on through life. You boys are so unique and so amazing in your own individual ways. Just know, with every fiber in your soul, how much your daddy loves you.

I simply feel that words can't truly capture what is in my heart. You are everything to me—just everything. I want to live a thousand more lifetimes with you. I really do. But that's not how it works.

So when I go, don't fear. I will always be near. I am forever with you, always will be.

You are the greatest sons a man could ever ask for.

Love,

Your Daddy

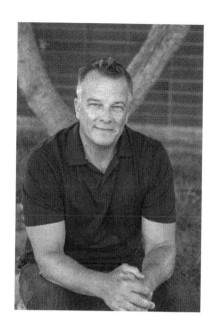

About the Author

Chris Meyer owns funeral homes. Prior to his career in the funeral industry, he wrote, directed, and produced an independent film in New York, then moved to Hollywood where he was a screenwriter.

More recently, he and a friend invented an anonymous loan search engine (and software) that educates and empowers all borrowers in their search for the best loan for their specific needs (www.MagillaLoans.com).

He grew up in Pleasantville, New York, attended Brandeis University and Vermont Law School, and now lives in Northern California with his wife of eighteen years and their three sons.

You will, most likely, find him on a field, or in a gym, coaching one of his sons' teams.

Made in the USA
San Bernardino, CA
20 January 2020